MEDICAL THINGS EXPLAINED

MTE

by Stacie the PA

Foot & Ankle Pain 101:

A Patient's Complete Guide to Symptoms, Treatments, and Prevention

By Stacie the PA

For permission requests, contact:
Medical Things Explained
Email: *medicalthingsexplained@gmail.com*

ISBN: 978-1-970376-03-6

Printed in the United States of America
First Edition, 2025

Cover design and layout by **Stacie the PA™**
Published by **Medical Things Explained / Stacie the PA / Bowker**

Disclaimer

This book is for educational purposes only and is not intended to replace professional medical advice, diagnosis, or treatment.

Foot and ankle problems can range from mild to serious, and many conditions require evaluation by a qualified healthcare professional such as an orthopedic surgeon, podiatrist, primary care provider, or other licensed clinician.

Always seek the advice of your medical provider with any questions you may have about your symptoms, diagnosis, imaging results, or treatment plan. Never disregard professional medical advice or delay seeking it because of something you have read in this book.

If you believe you may be experiencing a medical emergency—such as severe injury, inability to bear weight, loss of sensation, sudden color changes, signs of infection, or any other urgent concern—call 911 or your local emergency number immediately.

Medication names, brand names, and examples of products or supplements in this book are provided solely to help readers understand common treatment options. They do not represent endorsement by the author. Always consult your healthcare team before starting any new medication, supplement, exercise program, brace, orthotic, or home treatment.

Some links or products mentioned in this book may appear on the author's Amazon page as part of an affiliate partnership. If a purchase is made through those links, the author may receive a small commission at no additional cost to the reader. These partnerships help support the creation of future patient education materials.

Acknowledgement and Dedication

I would like to express my heartfelt gratitude to the many healthcare professionals I have had the privilege of learning from and working alongside throughout my career. From teachers and professors who built the foundation of my medical training to the clinicians and support staff who bring skill and compassion to every patient encounter—you have each shaped my understanding of medicine in meaningful, lasting ways.

During my residency and surgical training at Duke University Hospital, I learned the importance of precision, collaboration, and humility at the bedside and in the operating room. Later, as a practicing Physician Assistant, I had the opportunity to assist in a variety of orthopedic and lower extremity surgeries, working with multiple talented surgeons whose guidance continues to influence how I teach, write, and support patients today.

A special note of appreciation goes to Dr. Wade, whose expertise in foot and ankle surgery contributed valuable clinical insight to this book. I have had the privilege of operating with her—as well as with many skilled orthopedic surgeons over the years—and I remain grateful for the shared experiences that helped shape the practical, patient-centered approach of this guide.

Her input represents one viewpoint among many dedicated professionals who strive to improve patient care.

To my colleagues across medicine—physicians, physician assistants, nurse practitioners, nurses, anesthetists, pharmacists, therapists, social workers, radiology teams, surgical technologists, administrative staff, and ICU teams—thank you for your knowledge, mentorship, and tireless commitment to healing. Your teamwork and dedication continue to inspire me.

This book—and the entire Patient Education 101 series—is dedicated to all of you who serve, teach, and care with heart.

Thank you for reminding me every day that medicine, at its best, is both a science and an art.

How to use this book

Many patients tell me they leave their first office visit—no matter the specialty—feeling more confused than reassured. If that sounds familiar, this book is for you.

My goal is to help you understand what's happening in your body, feel prepared for your appointments, and feel more in control of your care.
— Stacie the PA

This book is designed to be a true workbook—something you can write in, underline, and return to whenever you need it.

Inside, you'll find:

- Short explanations written in plain language
- Simple drawings to make anatomy easy to understand
- Checklists and worksheets to help you stay organized
- Questions to ask your provider so you get the right information
- Blank sections where you can jot down notes, symptoms, or instructions

Here are a few ways to use this book:

- Write down where your pain is and how it changes
- Keep track of new symptoms or flare-ups
- Note what treatments help (and what don't)
- Record instructions from your provider, including medications, exercises, imaging, or follow-up plans

This book is your space to make sense of your symptoms, prepare for visits, and stay informed every step of the way.

✎ Notes:

Table of Contents

SECTION 1

Understanding Your Foot & Ankle

A simple guide to how your foot and ankle work and why pain develops.

Why Foot and Ankle Pain Is So Common

- Your feet and ankles work harder than almost any other part of your body.
- They carry all of your body weight every time you stand, walk, climb stairs, or run.
- Because they work so much and move in many different ways, they are easily stressed, irritated, or injured.
- Most experts, including the American Academy of Orthopaedic Surgeons (AAOS), explain that foot and ankle pain is common for a few main reasons:

1. A Lot of Moving Parts

Your foot has 26 bones, 33 joints, and more than 100 muscles, tendons, and ligaments.

That's a lot of parts working together in a small space.

When even one small part becomes irritated or injured, it can cause pain. For example:

- A tiny tendon can become inflamed.
- A small ligament can stretch or tear.
- A joint can become stiff or arthritic.

2. Your Feet Carry Your Whole Body

Every step you take puts pressure on your feet and ankles.

Doctors at Mayo Clinic explain that each step can place 1.5 to 2 times your body weight through the foot. When you run or jump, that pressure increases even more.

This constant pressure makes the foot and ankle more likely to:

- Get sore
- Develop overuse injuries
- Wear down over time

3. The Foot Must Be Strong and Flexible

Your foot has to do two opposite jobs:

- Stay strong and stable to support you when you stand
- Stay flexible so it can absorb shock when you walk or run

According to the Cleveland Clinic, this balance of strength and flexibility helps your foot work well, but it also makes the foot easier to injure. If one area becomes too tight, weak, or tired, it can throw off the whole system.

4. Many Injuries Happen During Normal Daily Activities

Foot and ankle injuries don't only happen in sports. Even small missteps can twist the ankle or strain a tendon. They often happen during simple activities like:

- Stepping off a curb
- Missing a stair
- Walking on uneven ground
- Wearing shoes that don't fit well

5. The Foot Works All Day With Very Little Rest

Unlike other body parts, your feet rarely get a break.
As Johns Hopkins Medicine notes, the foot is active from the moment you get out of bed until you lie down again at night.

This constant use can lead to:

- Overuse injuries
- Inflammation
- Tired muscles
- Stiff joints

6. Medical Conditions Can Affect the Feet

The foot is often the first place certain health problems show up. Some medical conditions make foot and ankle pain more likely.

Examples include:

- Arthritis
- Diabetes
- Nerve problems
- Poor circulation
- Flat feet or high arches

7. Small Problems Can Grow Quickly

Because the foot has so many moving parts, one small issue can lead to more problems. For example:

- A sprain can lead to swelling.
- Swelling can affect your balance.
- Poor balance can lead to more sprains.

In Summary: The Foot Takes a Long Time to Heal

- Your feet have many small joints, ligaments, and nerves.
- Every step places 2 to 4 times your body weight through the foot.
- Some tendons, like the Achilles, get poor blood flow.
- Swelling in the foot lasts longer because of gravity.
- Feet carry us all day—unlike wrist injuries that can rest completely.

Key Terms

- **Tendon**: The tissue that connects muscle to bone
- **Ligament**: The tissue that connects bone to bone
- **Joint**: Where two bones meet
- **Inflammation**: Swelling and irritation inside the body
- **Overuse**: Too much stress without enough rest

Footnote Summary

- Your feet carry your body all day.
- They have many small parts that can get irritated or injured.
- Everyday activities and medical conditions can cause problems.
- If your pain lasts more than 1 or 2 weeks, see a foot specialist.

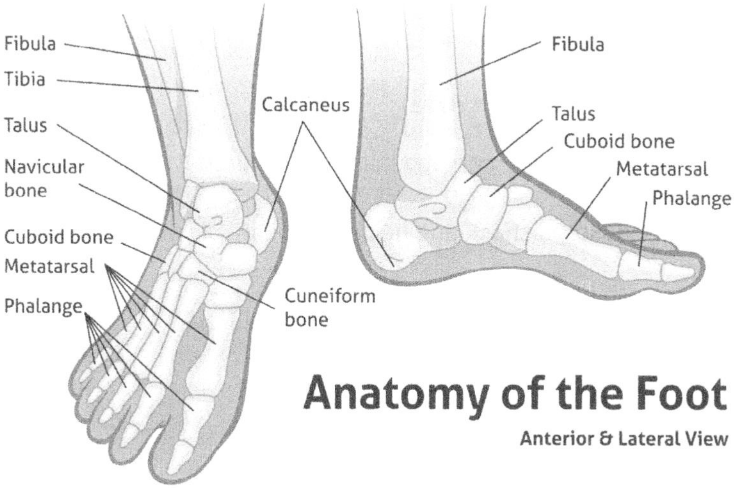

Bones of the Foot and Ankle

Your foot and ankle are made of many small bones that work together to help you stand, walk, and balance.

Doctors at the AAOS and Mayo Clinic explain that the foot has **26 bones**, and each one has a specific job.

When even one bone becomes irritated, broken, or out of alignment, it can cause pain.

To make things easier to understand, we divide the foot into **three main parts**:

1. The Hindfoot (Back of the Foot)

This area includes two strong bones:

- **Calcaneus (Heel Bone)** – This is the largest bone in the foot. It absorbs the impact every time your heel hits the ground. Injuries here often cause heel pain.
- **Talus** – This bone sits on top of the heel bone and forms the lower part of your ankle joint. It helps your ankle bend up and down.

2. The Midfoot (The Arch Area)

These bones form your arch and help keep your foot stable when you stand or walk.
The midfoot absorbs shock and helps you push off when you take a step.

The midfoot is the "bridge" of your foot and includes:

- **Navicular**
- **Cuboid**
- **Three cuneiform bones**

Pain in the midfoot often happens during:

- Walking on uneven ground
- Standing for long periods
- Wearing unsupportive shoes

3. The Forefoot (Front of the Foot)

Bunions, hammertoes, toe injuries, and nerve problems often affect the forefoot.

This area includes:

- **Metatarsals** – These are the five long bones at the front of the foot. They carry your body weight when you walk. Pain in these bones can feel like soreness in the ball of your foot.
- **Phalanges (Toes)** – Each toe has several small bones. They help with balance and push-off when you walk.

Notes:

The Ankle Joint

Your ankle is made of **three bones** that work together:

- **Tibia** — The main shin bone
- **Fibula** — The thinner bone on the outside of your leg
- **Talus** — This bone sits between the leg bones and the heel bone

These bones form a **hinge joint** that allows your foot to bend **up and down**. The joint also helps with **side-to-side balance**.

According to the AAOS, **ankle sprains** are one of the most common injuries because this joint does a lot of work and can twist easily.

When a bone is injured—even slightly—the entire foot can feel it.

These bones are important because they:

- Support your body weight
- Absorb shock
- Let you walk and run
- Help you stay balanced
- Protect important nerves, blood vessels, and tendons

Key Terms

- **Hindfoot**: The back of the foot (heel area)
- **Midfoot**: The arch area
- **Forefoot**: The toes and ball of the foot
- **Talus**: The ankle bone that helps you bend your foot
- **Metatarsals**: The long bones in the front of the foot

Notes:

Footnote Summary

- Your foot has **26 bones**.
- The **heel and ankle bones** support most of your weight.
- The **arch bones** help you stay balanced.
- The **front of your foot** helps you push off when walking.
- Even small bone problems can cause **big pain**.

Tendons, Ligaments, and Muscles

Your foot and ankle move because of **tendons, ligaments, and muscles** working together.

These soft tissues help you stand, walk, balance, and push off the ground.

When any of them become irritated, stretched, or torn, **foot and ankle pain** can begin quickly.

- **Muscles** create movement. They tighten and relax to move your foot and ankle.
- **Tendons** are strong cords that connect muscle to bone. They pull on bones to help you walk, run, and stay balanced.
- **Ligaments** connect bone to bone. They hold joints together and keep your ankle from **"rolling" too far.**

According to **the AAOS** and **Johns Hopkins**, the following tendons are the most commonly injured:

1. Achilles Tendon

- The strongest tendon in your body
- Connects your calf muscles to your heel
- Helps you walk, climb stairs, run, and jump

Achilles injuries often start with tightness or pain in the back of the ankle.

Common problems include:

- Tendonitis (irritation)
- Tendinosis (wear and tear)
- Partial or full tears

2. Posterior Tibial Tendon

- Runs along the inside of your ankle
- Supports your arch
- Keeps your foot from **"collapsing inward"**

This tendon is important for standing, walking, and balance.
When injured, you may develop:

- Flatfoot
- Swelling
- Pain along the inside of the foot

3. Peroneal Tendons

- Run along the outside of your ankle
- Help turn your foot outward
- Help prevent ankle sprains

When irritated, you may feel:

- Pain on the outside of the ankle
- Weakness during walking

4. Anterior Tibial Tendon

- Located on the front of the ankle
- Helps lift your foot up when you take a step

Injury may cause:

- Foot slapping
- Difficulty lifting the foot

5. Flexor and Extensor Tendons

These tendons help with **balance** and **pushing off the ground**. They move your toes:

- **Flexors** curl the toes
- **Extensors** lift the toes

Important Ligaments in the Foot and Ankle

Ligaments are strong bands of tissue that connect **bone to bone**. They help **stabilize joints** and prevent too much movement. In the foot and ankle, certain ligaments are especially important.

1. Lateral Ankle Ligaments (Outside of the Ankle)

Sprains often happen when the ankle rolls inward.
These are the most commonly injured ligaments.

They include:

- **ATFL** (anterior talofibular ligament)
- **CFL** (calcaneofibular ligament)

2. Deltoid Ligament (Inside of the Ankle)

This strong ligament helps keep your ankle stable.
Injuries here may cause:

- Pain on the inner side of the ankle
- Difficulty walking

3. Plantar Fascia

The **plantar fascia** is a thick band of tissue that runs along the bottom of the foot. It supports the arch and absorbs shock.

When irritated, it causes **heel pain** called **plantar fasciitis**.

Why These Structures Matter

According to **the Mayo Clinic** and **Cleveland Clinic**, tendons and ligaments:

- Provide stability
- Keep your foot aligned
- Help absorb shock
- Protect your bones and joints

Small injuries can lead to **big problems** because these tissues are used **all day, every day**.

Key Terms

- **Tendon**: Tissue that connects muscle to bone
- **Ligament**: Tissue that connects bone to bone
- **Achilles tendon**: Large tendon behind the ankle
- **ATFL / CFL**: Important ligaments on the outside of the ankle
- **Plantar fascia**: Tissue on the bottom of the foot that supports the arch

Notes:

Footnote Summary

- Muscles move your foot.
- Tendons connect muscle to bone.
- Ligaments connect bone to bone and keep joints stable.

Common problem areas include:

- The Achilles tendon
- The inside of the ankle
- The outside of the ankle
- Even small strains can cause pain because your foot works all day.

Nerves of the Foot

Your foot and ankle have several important **nerves**. These nerves allow you to feel **touch, pressure, temperature, and pain**. They also help control **muscle movement**.

According to experts at **Cleveland Clinic** and **Johns Hopkins**, nerve problems in the foot are **very common** and can cause:

- Tingling
- Burning
- Numbness
- Sharp pain

To keep it simple, your foot nerves can be grouped into **four main pathways**:

1. Tibial Nerve

The **tibial nerve** runs down the back of your leg and behind the inside of your ankle. It then splits into smaller branches that supply the bottom of your foot.

What it controls:

- Feeling on the bottom of the foot
- Movement of the toes
- Some arch control

Common problems:

- **Tarsal tunnel syndrome** (nerve is pinched near the inside of the ankle)
- Numbness or burning in the arch or bottom of the foot
- Tingling in the toes

2. Peroneal Nerves

The **peroneal nerves** wrap around the outside of the knee and travel down the outer side of the lower leg and ankle.

There are two branches:

Superficial peroneal nerve:

- Controls feeling on the top of the foot
- Helps the foot turn outward

Deep peroneal nerve:

- Controls feeling between the first and second toes
- Helps lift the foot

Common problems:

- Numbness on the top of the foot
- Weakness lifting the foot (**foot drop**)
- Pain or tingling on the outer ankle

3. Sural Nerve

The **sural nerve** travels along the back and outer side of the ankle. It controls **feeling on the outer foot and heel**.

Common problems:

- Burning or tingling on the outside of the foot
- Pain after ankle sprains or from wearing tight boots

4. Saphenous Nerve

The **saphenous nerve** runs along the **inner side** of the ankle and lower leg. It controls **feeling along the inner ankle and inner foot**.

Common problems:

- Numbness on the inner ankle
- Sensitivity after an injury or swelling

Why Foot Nerves Become Irritated

Foot nerves can become irritated for many reasons, including:

- Swelling from an injury
- Tight shoes
- Diabetes or high blood sugar
- Pressure on the nerve
- Arthritis
- Old ankle sprains
- Low back problems (such as **lumbar radiculopathy**)

Because these nerves travel through **tight spaces**, even mild swelling can press on the nerve and cause symptoms.

Notes:

CUTANEOUS INNERVATION OF THE FOOT

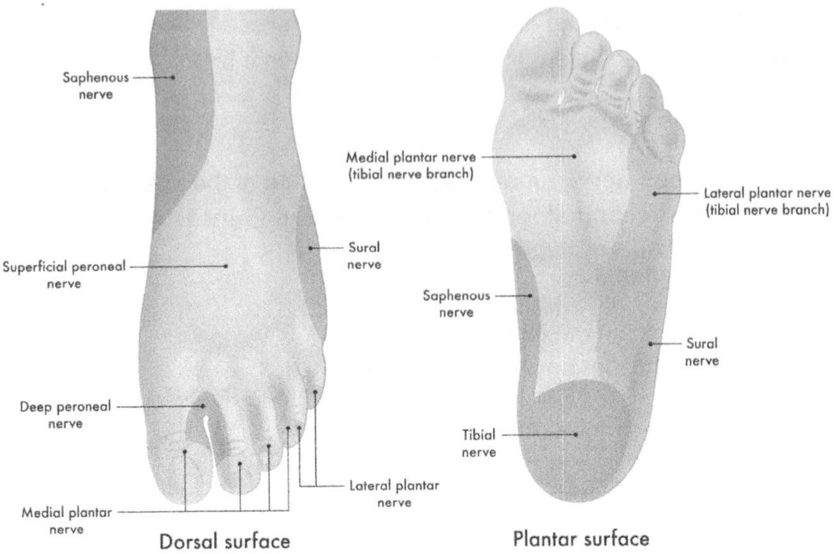

Symptoms of Nerve Irritation

Nerve problems often feel different than **bone, tendon, or muscle problems**.

Common symptoms of nerve irritation include:

- Tingling (a "pins and needles" feeling)
- Burning
- Electric-shock sensations
- Numbness
- Sharp, shooting pains
- Hot or cold sensations
- Feeling like your sock is **"bunched up"**, even when it isn't

If these symptoms **last longer than 2 weeks**, they should be **checked by a medical provider**.

Key Terms

- **Nerve**: Sends signals for feeling and movement
- **Tingling**: A "pins and needles" feeling
- **Tarsal tunnel**: A tight space on the inside of the ankle where a nerve can get pinched
- **Neuropathy**: Nerve irritation or damage
- **Foot drop**: Trouble lifting the foot, often caused by nerve weakness

Footnote Summary

- Your foot has several **nerves** that control **feeling** and **movement**.
- The **tibial nerve** affects the **bottom** of the foot.
- The **peroneal nerves** affect the **top** and **outside** of the foot.
- Numbness, burning, or tingling can mean a **nerve is irritated**.
- Lasting nerve symptoms should be **checked by a medical provider**.

Notes:

Movements of the Foot and Ankle

Your foot and ankle can move in many different ways. These movements help you:

- Stand
- Balance
- Walk
- Run
- Change direction

According to **the AAOS** and **Mayo Clinic**, each movement is controlled by specific **muscles** and **tendons**. When one type of movement becomes painful, it can give **clues about which tendon, ligament, or joint may be injured**.

Here are the **main movements** your foot and ankle can do:

1. Dorsiflexion (Foot Up)

This is when you **lift your foot upward**, like when taking your foot off the gas pedal.

Used for:

- Walking
- Climbing stairs
- Keeping your balance

Main muscle/tendon involved: Anterior tibial tendon (on the front of the ankle)

Pain here may mean:

- Tendon irritation
- Ankle arthritis
- Tight calf muscles

2. Plantarflexion (Foot Down)

This is when you **point your toes downward**, like pressing on a gas pedal.

Used for:

- Walking and running
- Jumping
- Standing on your toes

Main muscle/tendon involved: Achilles tendon

Pain here may mean:

- Achilles tendonitis
- Tight calf muscles
- Tendon wear and tear

3. Inversion (Foot Turns Inward)

This is when the **sole of your foot turns toward your other foot**.

Used for:

- Balancing
- Changing direction

Main structures involved: Inner ankle ligaments and **posterior tibial tendon**

Pain here may mean:

- Ankle sprain
- Tendon strain
- Flatfoot problems

4. Eversion (Foot Turns Outward)

This is when the **sole of your foot turns away** from your other foot.

Used for:

- Side-to-side movements
- Walking on uneven ground

Main structures involved: Peroneal tendons (along the outside of the ankle)

Pain here may mean:

- Peroneal tendonitis
- Outer ankle sprain
- Instability from past injuries

5. Toe Flexion (Curling Toes Down)

This is when your **toes curl downward** toward the floor.

Used for:

- Pushing off when walking
- Balancing on uneven ground

Main structures involved: Flexor tendons

Pain here may mean:

- Tendon irritation
- Hammertoe changes
- Nerve irritation

6. Toe Extension (Lifting Toes Up)

This is when your **toes lift upward** toward your shin.

Used for:

- Walking
- Running
- Balance

Main structures involved: Extensor tendons

Pain here may mean:

- Tendon irritation
- Pressure from tight shoes
- Nerve irritation between the toes

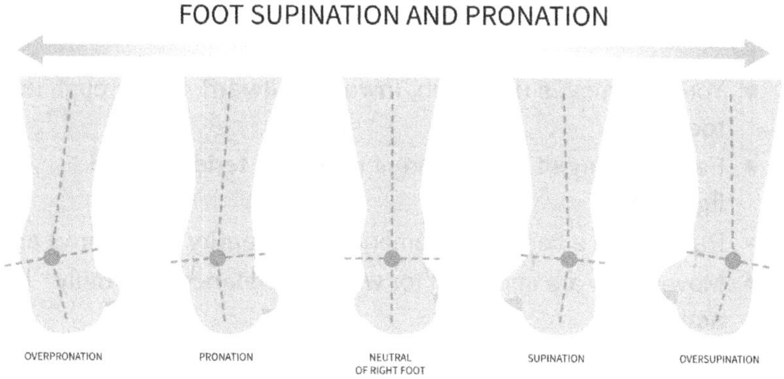

How Movement Helps Identify Injury

Pain with a specific motion can help identify **which part of the foot is irritated**. This is why your provider may ask you to move your foot in different ways during an exam.

For example:

- **Pain when lifting the foot** → front ankle tendons
- **Pain when pointing the toes** → Achilles tendon
- **Pain when turning the foot inward** → inner ankle ligaments
- **Pain when turning the foot outward** → outer ankle ligaments or peroneal tendons

Understanding how movement relates to pain can help **locate the injury** more accurately.

Key Terms

- **Dorsiflexion**: Foot lifts upward
- **Plantarflexion**: Foot points downward
- **Inversion**: Foot turns inward
- **Eversion**: Foot turns outward
- **Flexion / Extension**: Toes curl (flexion) or lift (extension)

Footnote Summary

- Your foot moves **up, down, inward, outward**, and through the **toes**.
- Each movement uses different **muscles**, **tendons**, and **ligaments**.
- Pain during a certain movement helps **identify the injured area**.
- Movements are important for **walking**, **balance**, and **daily activities**.

Notes:

Women's Joint Health

Menopause can cause:

- Joint pain
- Tendon irritation
- Foot stiffness

This is part of a condition called **musculoskeletal menopause syndrome**.

According to experts, **estrogen replacement is now considered safer for many women when medically appropriate.**

However, **walking is not enough** to protect joints. Women need:

- **Weight-bearing exercise**
- **Strength training**
- **Stair climbing**
- **Core strengthening**

These activities help protect your **bones**, **tendons**, and **balance** as estrogen levels drop.

Notes:

Acute vs. Chronic Ankle and Foot Pain

Foot and ankle pain can come on suddenly or build up slowly over time. Knowing the difference helps you understand **what may be wrong** and **when to see a medical provider**.

Acute Pain (New Pain)

Acute pain starts suddenly—often after an injury. It is your body's **alarm system**, warning you that something may be:

- Stretched
- Sprained
- Torn

Most mild injuries begin to **improve within a few days**.

Common causes of acute pain:

- Rolling your ankle
- Stepping wrong
- Missing a stair
- A direct hit or fall

Symptoms of acute pain:

- Swelling
- Bruising
- Warmth
- Trouble walking
- Tender spots

When to Seek Care

If your pain is **not improving within 2–3 weeks**, specialists recommend getting it evaluated.

The ankle has many small **ligaments**, **tendons**, and **joints**. Even a **"simple sprain"** can hide a deeper problem that needs attention.

Don't wait months or years to get ankle or foot pain checked.

- Early evaluation = faster diagnosis and shorter recovery
- Waiting too long = harder treatment and possible need for advanced care

Chronic Pain (Long-Lasting Pain)

Chronic pain lasts more than **4–6 weeks**, even with rest and home care.

This type of pain may:

- Come and go
- Feel worse after activity
- Cause stiffness
- Make your foot or ankle feel weak

Common Causes of Chronic Pain

- Tendon problems
- Old injuries that didn't heal fully
- Arthritis
- Nerve problems
- Repeated sprains
- Flat feet or high arches

Long-lasting pain should be evaluated by a medical provider. Early treatment can help **prevent future problems**. These symptoms may point to a more serious injury that needs attention.

Notes:

Red Flags — When to Call Right Away

Call a doctor or go to urgent care if you notice:

- **Severe swelling**
- A **bone that looks "off"** or out of place
- **Inability to put weight** on the foot
- **Numbness, tingling, or cold toes**
- **Signs of infection** (fever, redness, or spreading warmth)

These may be signs of a **medical emergency**.

Key Terms

- **Acute**: New or sudden
- **Chronic**: Lasting weeks or longer
- **Sprain**: A stretched or torn ligament
- **Strain**: An injured muscle or tendon
- **Inflammation**: Swelling and irritation inside the body

Footnote Summary

- **Acute pain** starts suddenly and usually improves within a few days.
- **Chronic pain** lasts more than 4–6 weeks and may mean something isn't healing.
- If pain lasts more than **1–2 weeks without getting better**, get it checked.
- **Call right away** for severe swelling, numbness, or trouble walking.

SECTION 2

Preparing for Your Visit

What to think about before your appointment so you get the most out of your care.

Before Your Visit: What to Think About

- During your visit, you may be asked **many questions in a short amount of time.**
  Thinking about your answers **ahead of time** can help both **you and your medical team.**
- These are simple things to think about before you see your **foot and ankle specialist.**
  They will help you **remember the most important details about your pain.**

What to Bring to Your Visit

Bring:

- Any **old X-rays**, **MRIs**, or **doctor notes**
- **Shoe inserts**, braces, or walking aids you've used
- A **list of treatments** you've already tried

Diagnosis is a **step-by-step process**. Starting from scratch takes longer, even for second opinions.

A second opinion still requires:

- **Your full records**
- Or updated testing, if records are missing

Having the **prior opinion** helps:

- Rule out certain problems faster
- Speed up the path to getting answers
- Even if the answer isn't what you hoped for, it's better to know early

Describing Your Pain

Use **one finger** to point to where the pain is. **Don't use your whole hand**—this makes it harder to identify the source. Pain described as **"all over"** is not helpful for diagnosis.

Be ready to answer these questions:

- Is the pain always in the same spot?
- Does it move, or does it stay in one area?
- Does it hurt when you stand up from sitting?
- Where exactly does it hurt when you walk?

These answers help us find the **true pain generator**—the structure that's really causing your symptoms.

Notes:

What Your Surgeon Wishes You Knew

These are simple truths your foot and ankle surgeon **wants you to remember**—based on years of seeing patients, treating injuries, and guiding recovery.

- **Early care = easier care**
  Surgeon's Note: *"Catching foot problems early saves people months of frustration."*
- **Pain doesn't mean "stop everything"—but adjust**
  Movement helps recovery. Modify your activity, don't eliminate it completely.
- **Healing takes time**
  Especially with tendons, ligaments, and nerves. Be patient with your body.
- **Imaging is only part of the picture**
  MRIs and X-rays don't show everything. ***Surgeon's Note:*** *"The exam often tells us more than the MRI.*
- **Most bumps aren't dangerous**
  Not every lump or swelling is a sign of serious damage. But new or rapidly changing masses should be checked
- **Strength matters more as you age**
  Strong muscles support your joints, reduce pain, and prevent injuries.
- **Walking alone is not enough exercise**
  You also need balance training, stretching, and strength exercises.
- **Shoes matter more than people think**
  Poor footwear can cause or worsen foot and ankle problems.
- **Pain doesn't always match the picture**
  A severe-looking scan might not hurt, while a normal scan might. Pain is complex.
- **Surgery is teamwork**
  Your effort after surgery is just as important as the surgeon's work in the operating room.
- **Kindness helps everyone**
  Recovery is hard. A kind attitude toward yourself, your care team, and others makes a difference.

Notes:

Questions to Think About Before Your Visit

Surgeon's Note: *"Clear details help us find the real source of the pain."*

1. Where is your pain? (Think about the exact spot.
Is it the inside of the ankle, the outside, the heel, the top of the foot, the bottom, or the toes?)

____

____

____

____

2. When did the pain start? (Was it today, a few days ago, a few weeks ago, or longer?

____

Did it begin suddenly or slowly?

____

____

3. Did something cause your pain?

____

____

Try to remember if you:

- ☐ Twisted your ankle
- ☐ Stepped wrong
- ☐ Fell
- ☐ Started a new activity
- ☐ Wore new or different shoes
- ☐ Or if it started for no clear reason. –

4. What does it feel like? Sharp? Aching? Burning? Tingling?
Knowing the "feeling" helps your provider understand the cause.

____

____

____

____

5. What makes it worse? Walking, standing, stairs, first steps in the morning, exercise, certain shoes?

6. What makes it better? Rest, ice, heat, elevation, new shoes, stretching, medications?

7. How much does the pain affect your day? Does it change how you walk, work, sleep, or move?

8. Can you walk normally? Do you limp or avoid putting weight on the foot?

9. Have you had this pain before? If yes, think about what helped last time.

10. Are you having any concerning symptoms?

Such as:

- ☐ Swelling
- ☐ Bruising
- ☐ Numbness
- ☐ Tingling
- ☐ Cold toes
- ☐ Redness
- ☐ A feeling of weakness or "giving way"

  These details help your provider decide if you need imaging or special care.

Daily Activity Questions to Think About

1. What shoes do you usually wear? Supportive shoes, sandals, boots, or mostly barefoot?

____

____

____

2. Do you stand or sit a lot? Your daily routine affects ankle and foot pain.

____

____

3. Have you already tried anything to help? Ice, rest, braces, inserts, medications, stretching?

____

____

____

____

____

____

____

____

Questions You May Want to Ask Your Provider

Bring this list with you. Add your own questions as needed.

- ☐ What is my diagnosis?
- ☐ What is causing this pain?
- ☐ Is there anything I should avoid doing?
- ☐ What can I do at home to help it heal?
- ☐ Do I need imaging (X-ray, ultrasound, MRI)?
- ☐ What treatment do you recommend first?
- ☐ How long should I expect recovery to take?
- ☐ When should I follow up?
- ☐ When should I call if something changes?
- ☐ Will I need physical therapy?
- ☐ What shoes or inserts do you recommend?

Notes:

In Summary:

Before Your Visit

Bring this filled-out page to your visit. It helps your provider understand your pain and treat it more effectively.

- Be specific about **where it hurts** and what makes it **better or worse**
- Write down **how long** the pain has been present
- Add your own **questions**, so you feel ready and informed

During the Exam

Most foot and ankle exams are:

- **Simple**
- **Gentle**
- **Quick** (usually just a few minutes)

Your provider may:

- Look at your foot and ankle
- Press gently on different areas (palpation)
- Move your foot to check its range of motion
- Watch how you walk (gait exam)
- Examine your shoes for wear or fit

Imaging (Only If Needed)

Many foot and ankle problems can be diagnosed **without imaging**, but pictures may help confirm the diagnosis. If needed, your provider may recommend:

- **X-ray** – to check bones, alignment, and arthritis
- **Ultrasound** – to look at tendons or fluid buildup
- **MRI** – to assess ligaments, tendons, cartilage, or stress fractures

Key Terms

- **Palpation**: Gently pressing to find tender spots
- **Range of motion**: How far a joint can move
- **Gait**: The way you walk
- **Numbness**: Decreased or lost feeling
- **Tenderness**: Pain when an area is touched

Imaging Tests Explained

Imaging helps your provider understand what may be causing your pain. These tests help show the **bones**, **joints**, **tendons**, **ligaments**, and **soft tissues** inside your foot.

Not every patient needs imaging. Many foot and ankle problems can be diagnosed with a simple physical exam. But when pictures are helpful, these are the **most commonly used tests**:

X-ray (Radiograph)

What it is: An X-ray uses a small amount of radiation to take pictures of your bones.

What it shows:

- Broken bones (**fractures**)
- Arthritis
- Bone spurs
- Bone alignment
- Joint spacing

Why it's used: It is usually the **first test ordered** because it's:

- Quick
- Painless
- Good for showing bone details

What it does *not* show well:

- Tendons
- Ligaments
- Nerves
- Muscles

MRI (Magnetic Resonance Imaging)

What it is: A MRI uses **magnets** (not radiation) to make detailed pictures of **soft tissues**.

What it shows:

- Tendons (including tears or swelling)
- Ligaments
- Cartilage
- Muscles
- Stress fractures
- Nerve irritation
- Inflammation

Why it's used: MRI gives the **clearest picture** of soft tissue injuries that can't be seen on an X-ray.

Good for:

- Achilles tendon problems
- Tendon tears
- Ankle sprains that will not heal
- Stress fractures
- Plantar fasciitis that isn't improving

Notes:

Ultrasound (US)

What it is: Ultrasound uses **sound waves** to look at tissues **in real time**.

What it shows:

- Tendons
- Ligaments
- Fluid or swelling
- Cysts
- Motion of tendons as you move your foot

Why it's used: Ultrasound is **quick, painless**, and can show problems **while your foot is moving**.

Good for:

- Achilles tendon problems
- Plantar fasciitis
- Nerve irritation
- Fluid around tendons

CT Scan (Computed Tomography)

What it is: A CT scan is a special type of X-ray that takes **many images at once** to create a **3D picture**.

What it shows:

- Complex fractures
- Bone detail
- Joint alignment
- Bone cysts or tumors (rare)

Why it's used: CT is helpful when your provider needs to see **fine bone detail** or **plan for surgery**.

Good for:

- Hard-to-see fractures
- Ankle arthritis evaluation
- Foot deformities
- Surgical planning or mapping

Bone Scan *(Less Common)*

What it is:
A small amount of **tracer** is injected into your bloodstream. A special camera then looks for **"hot spots"** in the bones.

What it shows:

- Stress fractures
- Infections
- Bone inflammation

Why it's used: Bone scans are used **less often**, but may help when **other tests are unclear**.

Nerve Tests (EMG or Nerve Conduction Study)

What they are: Tests that check how well your **nerves send signals** to your muscles.

What they show:

- Nerve irritation
- Nerve compression
- Whether pain is coming from the **lower back** (such as lumbar radiculopathy)

Good for:

- Tingling
- Numbness
- Burning sensations
- Suspected nerve-related issues

Weight-Bearing Imaging

Some **X-rays** and **CT scans** may be done while **standing (weight-bearing).**

Why it's done: Many foot and ankle problems only show up **when you put weight on your foot**.

This helps diagnose:

- Flatfoot
- Arch collapse
- Arthritis
- Alignment problems

Which Imaging Test Might You Need?

Your provider will choose the right test based on:

- Your **symptoms**
- Your **exam**
- How **long** the pain has lasted
- Whether you had an **injury**
- If there is **swelling** or **nerve involvement**

Most patients start with an X-ray.
An MRI or ultrasound may be added **only if needed.**

Notes:

Why Imaging Doesn't Always Show the Pain

- An MRI may look normal, even when the source of pain is present but subtle.
- **X-rays** do not show tendons or ligaments
- Pain may come from **more than one source**
- **Nerve pain** often doesn't show up on imaging
- **Function** (how the foot works) matters more than just the picture

Key Terms

- **Radiograph**: A standard X-ray
- **Soft tissue**: Muscles, tendons, and ligaments
- **Stress fracture**: A tiny crack in the bone
- **Nerve conduction study**: A test that measures how nerves send signals
- **Weight-bearing**: Standing during the imaging test

Footnote Summary

- **X-rays** show bones
- **MRI** shows tendons, ligaments, and soft tissue
- **Ultrasound** shows tendons, fluid, and motion
- **CT** provides highly detailed images of bones
- **Nerve tests** help diagnose tingling, numbness, and burning
- **Most patients begin with a simple X-ray**

Notes:

Checklist: What to Bring to Your First Visit

✔ 1. Photo ID and Insurance Card

- Driver's license or state ID
- Your current insurance card(s)

✔ 2. A List of Your Medications

Include:

- Prescription medications
- Over-the-counter medicines (ibuprofen, Tylenol, etc.)
- Vitamins and supplements
- Any recent changes to doses

✔ 3. Your Past Medical Records (if available)

Bring anything related to foot or ankle pain:

- Prior X-rays, MRI, or CT scans (reports + actual images if you have a CD/USB)
- Recent lab results
- Notes from your primary care provider or previous specialists
- EMG/Nerve tests (if you've had them)

✔ 4. A Timeline of Your Symptoms

Make a short note of:

- When your pain started
- What makes it better or worse
- Any injuries or changes in activity
- Whether the pain is constant or comes and goes

Notes:

✔ 5. Photos of Your Foot or Ankle

If your symptoms change through the day, bring:

- Pictures of swelling
- Bruising
- Skin changes
- Deformities (like bunions or hammertoes)

(Taken on your phone is perfectly fine.)

✔ 6. Your Shoes

Bring:

- The shoes you wear most often
- Any inserts or orthotics
  Providers often check shoe wear patterns to understand your gait.

✔ 7. Activity Information

Make a quick list of:

- Your job and daily standing/walking time
- Your exercise routine
- Any recent increase in mileage or training (if you are active or a runner)

✔ 8. A List of Treatments You've Already Tried. Include:

- Ice, heat
- Braces, boots, or splints
- Stretching or exercises
- Physical therapy
- Injections or medications

This helps avoid repeating things that didn't work.

✔ 9. Your Pain and Function Notes

Include:

- Where the pain is located
- How severe it is (0–10 scale)
- What daily activities are affected (walking, stairs, work, sleep)

✔ 10. Support Person (Optional)

Bring someone if you:

- Have difficulty walking
- Need help remembering instructions
- Feel anxious about medical visits

Notes:

Foot Myths

Many common beliefs about foot and ankle pain are **not true**. Believing these myths can lead to **delayed treatment, longer recovery, or worse injuries**.

Myth: "I should wait until it hurts really badly before coming in."

Fact: Early treatment prevents longer recovery times. Foot problems are **easier to treat** when caught early.

Myth: "If I can walk on it, it's not broken."

Fact: Many people walk on fractures without realizing it. **Walking does not rule out a break.**

Myth: "I can fix this with the right shoe alone."

Fact: Good shoes help, but they **do not replace** medical care, stretching, strengthening, or therapy.

Myth: "Rest will cure everything."

Fact: Rest helps **in the beginning**, but too much rest can cause:

- Stiffness
- Weakness
- Slower healing

Notes:

💤 Myth: "If I rest long enough, it will eventually go away."

Fact: Rest helps at first, but too much rest **weakens your muscles and tendons**. Most foot problems get better with:

- A mix of rest and movement
- Stretching
- Strengthening
- Supportive shoes
- Activity changes

🦶 Myth: "Pain in my toes means the problem is in my toes."

Fact: Toe pain often comes from **somewhere else**—like:

- The midfoot
- Nerves on the top of the foot
- Even the lower back. Pain isn't always felt where it starts.

💪 Myth: "If I keep walking through the pain, I'll 'toughen it up.'"

Fact: Pushing through pain can **turn a small injury into a big one**. Pain is your body's signal to:

- Adjust
- Protect
- Or get evaluated. **It is not something to ignore.**

Notes:

Notes:

SECTION 3

Common Ankle & Foot Conditions

Easy-to-understand explanations of the most frequent causes of pain.

A. Ligaments and Injury

Introduction

This chapter explains the **most common ankle and foot conditions** in clear, simple language. Each section tells you:

- What the condition is
- Why it happens
- What you can do at home
- When to see a specialist

We'll begin with injuries to the **ligaments and joints**—problems that often happen **suddenly**, like sprains or twists.

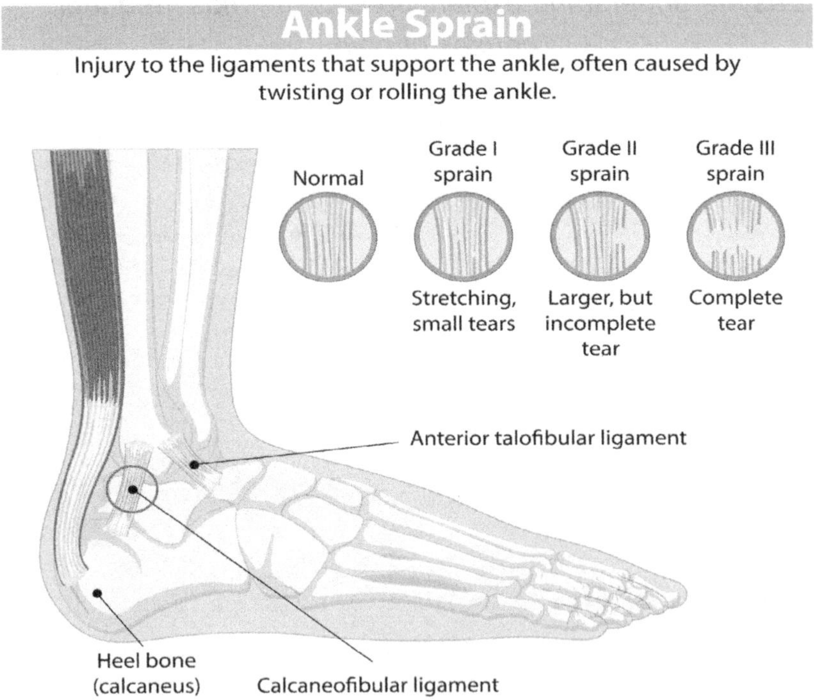

Ankle Sprains

What Are They?

An **ankle sprain** happens when the **ligaments** in your ankle are **stretched or torn**. Ligaments are strong bands of tissue that **hold the ankle bones together** and **keep the joint stable**.

Most sprains affect the **outside of the ankle**, where the ligaments are **thinner and more likely to be injured**.

Sprains can range from:

- **Mild**: Stretched ligament
- **Moderate**: Partial tear
- **Severe**: Complete tear with swelling and difficulty walking

Why Do They Happen?

Ankle sprains usually happen when the foot rolls inward, which stretches or tears the ligaments on the outside of the ankle.

Common causes include:

- Stepping off a curb wrong
- Tripping
- Landing on the side of your foot
- Wearing unsupportive shoes
- Sudden twisting during sports

You may be more likely to sprain your ankle if:

- Your ankle muscles are weak
- You've had previous sprains
- Your balance is poor
- You walk on uneven surfaces often

What Can You Do at Home?

Most **mild sprains** get better with simple home care.

1. RICE (First 1–3 Days)

- **Rest**: Avoid painful activity
- **Ice**: Apply 15–20 minutes at a time, several times a day
- **Compression**: Use an elastic bandage (not too tight)
- **Elevation**: Keep the ankle raised above heart level

---

2. Switch to MEAT (After 48–72 Hours)

- **Movement**: Gentle ankle circles, drawing the alphabet with your foot
- **Exercise**: Begin light strengthening as tolerated
- **Analgesics**: Use acetaminophen or NSAIDs (if safe for you)
- **Treatment**: Light stretching and supportive shoes

3. Protect the Ankle

- Wear a brace or elastic wrap for extra support
- Avoid uneven ground
- Take short walking breaks to avoid stiffness

---

4. Begin Gentle Exercises as Pain Improves

Exercises help prevent **future sprains**:

- Toe raises
- Ankle circles
- Towel scrunches
- Balance exercises (e.g., standing on one foot)

When to Seek Care

See a Specialist Right Away if You Have:

- Severe swelling
- A foot or ankle that looks "off" or crooked
- Inability to put any weight on the foot
- Numbness or tingling
- Blue or cold toes

See a Specialist Within 1–2 Weeks if:

- Pain is not improving
- You keep rolling or twisting the ankle
- It feels unstable or weak
- You cannot return to normal walking
- Swelling lasts more than 7–10 days

You May Need Imaging if:

- Pain is directly on the bone
- Walking is very difficult
- You heard a **"pop"** during the injury
- Pain lasts longer than expected

MRI may be ordered to check for:

- Torn ligaments
- Tendon injuries
- Hidden (**occult**) fractures
- Cartilage damage

Key Terms

- **Inversion**: When the ankle rolls inward
- **Ligament**: Tissue that connects one bone to another
- **Sprain**: A stretched or torn ligament
- **RICE**: Rest, Ice, Compression, Elevation
- **MEAT**: Movement, Exercise, Analgesics, Treatment

Footnote Summary

- A **sprain** is a **stretched or torn ligament**.
- Most sprains happen when the **ankle rolls inward**.
- Start with **RICE**, then switch to gentle movement after 2–3 days.
- **Seek care** if pain is severe, walking is difficult, or it's not improving within 1–2 weeks.
- **Early treatment** helps prevent **chronic ankle instability**.

Notes:

Chronic Ankle Instability

What Is It?

Chronic ankle instability means your ankle feels **weak**, **unstable**, or like it might **"give out,"** especially when walking on uneven ground. It often happens after **repeated ankle sprains**, or after **one sprain that never healed fully**.

People with chronic ankle instability may feel:

- **Wobbly or unsteady**
- **Pain on the outside of the ankle**
- **Frequent "rolling" of the ankle**
- **Swelling that comes and goes**

Why It Happens:

Chronic ankle instability usually occurs because the **ligaments on the outside of the ankle** became **stretched or torn** and never regained full strength.

Each sprain weakens the ligaments more, making future sprains more likely.

Common reasons include:

- Not healing fully after a sprain
- Repeated sprains over time
- Weak ankle or foot muscles
- Balance problems
- Wearing unsupportive shoes
- High arches or flat feet
- Loose ligaments from birth (**hypermobile joints**)

Notes:

What You Can Do at Home

Strength and **balance** play a major role in healing this condition.

1. **Wear a supportive brace**
   An ankle brace can help prevent the ankle from rolling again.
2. **Strengthen the ankle muscles**
   Exercises that help:
   • *Calf raises*
   • *Toe raises*
   • *Resistance band foot exercises*
   • *Ankle circles*
3. **Improve balance**
   Balance is one of the best ways to prevent repeat sprains. Try:
   • *Standing on one foot*
   • *Standing on a folded towel*
   • *Gentle wobble board exercises* (if safe for you)
4. **Use supportive shoes**
   Avoid worn-out shoes or flimsy sandals. Choose shoes that:
   • *Fit well*
   • *Hold the heel firmly*
   • *Provide arch support*
5. **RICE for flare-ups**
   If your ankle becomes sore or swollen after activity, **rest and ice** can help.

Notes:

When to Seek Care

Right away if:

- Your ankle keeps giving out
- You cannot walk safely
- You have weakness or numbness

Within a few weeks if:

- You continue to roll your ankle
- Pain or swelling returns often
- You feel unstable during daily activities
- Home exercises are not helping

Your provider may recommend:

- **Physical therapy**
- **Bracing**
- **Custom orthotics**
- **MRI** to check for ligament tears, tendon injuries, or cartilage problems

If instability is **severe** or **long-lasting**, **surgery** may be needed to repair or tighten loose ligaments.

Key Terms

- **Instability:** feeling like the joint might give out
- **Ligament:** tissue that holds bones together
- **Hypermobile:** extra loose joints
- **Balance training:** exercises that improve ankle control
- **Recurrent sprain:** sprains that keep happening

Notes:

Footnote Summary

- Chronic ankle instability is a **weak or wobbly ankle** after repeated sprains
- **Weak ligaments** and **poor balance** are common causes
- **Strengthening, balance exercises, bracing, and good shoes** can help
- **See a provider** if your ankle keeps rolling or doesn't feel stable

Notes:

Stress Fractures

What Are They?

A **stress fracture** is a tiny crack in a bone caused by **repeated stress or overuse**, not a single injury. They often occur in the **metatarsals** (front of the foot), **heel**, or **outer edge** of the foot.

Common symptoms:

- Sharp pain that gets worse with activity, better with rest
- Swelling or tenderness in one specific spot
- Pain with long walks or standing
- Trouble walking without limping

Stress fractures often start as **mild soreness** and **worsen over time**.

Why It Happens

According to AAOS and Mayo Clinic, stress fractures occur when **bones are overused** faster than they can rebuild.

More common in:

- Athletes, runners, dancers
- People who stand all day
- Military recruits
- People with **low bone density** or poor nutrition

Common causes include:

- Sudden increase in activity
- High-impact sports or hard surfaces
- Worn-out or unsupportive shoes
- Flat feet or high arches
- Low vitamin D or low calcium levels
- Returning to activity too soon after rest

What You Can Do at Home

1. **Stop painful activities.** Avoid running, jumping, or long walks.

2. **Apply ice.** 15–20 minutes to the painful area, especially after use.

3. **Wear supportive shoes.** Avoid thin or worn-out shoes. Look for:
   - *Cushion*
   - *Arch support*
   - *Firm heel*

4. **Switch to low-impact exercise.** Try:
   - *Swimming*
   - *Cycling*
   - *Upper-body workouts*

5. **Elevate the foot.** Use pillows to reduce swelling when resting.

6. **Use MEAT as pain improves**
   - *Movement* (gentle)
   - *Exercise* (as tolerated)
   - *Analgesics* (if safe)
   - *Treatment* (warm compresses later)

When to Seek Care

- Pain lasts more than **5–7 days**
- Pain is **severe or worsening**
- Limping or unable to walk
- Swelling that won't go down
- Tenderness over **one pinpoint spot**
- Recent increase in activity

Notes:

Your provider may recommend:

- **X-rays** (may not show early fractures)
- **MRI** (more accurate for early stress fractures)
- **Walking boot** or **activity change**
- **Vitamin D/calcium testing**
- **Orthotics or shoe inserts**

Most stress fractures **heal in 6–8 weeks** with proper care.

Decision Tree – Sprain vs. Something More

Did you roll your ankle outward (inversion injury)?
→ **Yes** → Most likely an ankle sprain
→ **No** → Consider other causes

Can you put weight on it?
→ **Yes** → Likely a sprain; try home care
→ **No** → Possible fracture — needs imaging

Is the swelling mostly on the outside of the ankle?
→ **Yes** → Typical lateral ankle sprain
→ **No** → Pain inside the ankle may mean a more serious injury

Is pain worse after 3–5 days?
→ **Yes** → May need evaluation for a deeper injury
→ **No** → Continue RICE, brace, and gentle movement

Notes:

Stress Fracture vs. Sprain

Stress Fracture	Sprain
Pain builds slowly over time	Pain happens suddenly
Very specific pain spot	Pain spread across ankle
Worse with activity, better with rest	Swelling and bruising appear quickly
Pain during activity	Pain when bearing weight
Pinpoint tenderness on bone	Tenderness around ligaments
Needs imaging to confirm	Often improves with home care

In Summary:

- *Ligament injuries and stress fractures are common foot and ankle problems.*
- *Sprains happen suddenly and usually heal with **rest, support, and therapy**.*
- *Stress fractures build slowly and need **rest and protective care** to heal.*
- *If pain lasts more than **1–2 weeks** or **you can't walk normally**, get checked to avoid long-term problems.*

Key Terms

- **Low-impact exercise:** Gentle activities that reduce stress on the foot, such as swimming or cycling
- **Metatarsals:** The long bones in the front (ball) of the foot
- **MRI:** An imaging test that can detect early stress fractures and soft-tissue changes
- **Stress fracture:** A tiny crack in a bone caused by repeated stress or overuse
- **Tenderness:** Pain felt when pressing on a small area of the foot

Footnote Summary

- A **stress fracture** is a tiny bone crack caused by overuse
- Pain gets **worse with activity** and better with **rest**
- **Supportive shoes**, **ice**, and **early care** help healing
- **Seek care** if pain lasts more than a week or walking is difficult

Notes:

B. Tendons

Intro: Next are tendon problems. Tendons connect muscles to bones and help you move your foot and ankle. When tendons get irritated or overworked, they can cause pain, swelling, or trouble walking.

Achilles Tendonitis / Tendinosis

What Is It?

The **Achilles tendon** is the strong band of tissue that connects your **calf muscles to your heel**. It helps you **walk**, **run**, **climb stairs**, and **stand on your toes**.

- **Tendonitis** means the tendon is **irritated and inflamed**
- **Tendinosis** means the tendon has **wear and tear** over time and becomes **thickened or stiff**

You may feel:

- Pain or stiffness in the back of your heel or ankle
- Swelling or warmth
- Pain when walking or climbing stairs
- Morning stiffness
- Tenderness when pressing on the tendon

Why It Happens

Achilles problems often come from **overuse** or **tight calf muscles**, even without a specific injury.

Common causes include:

- Sudden increase in activity
- Running on hills or hard surfaces
- Tight calves
- Poorly supportive shoes
- Flat feet or high arches
- Aging (tendons weaken with time)

What You Can Do at Home

1. **Rest the tendon.** Avoid running, jumping, hills, or long walks. *Gentle walking is okay if pain-free.*

2. **Ice the area.** Use ice for **15–20 minutes**, especially after activity.

3. **Wear supportive shoes**
   Look for:
   - *Good heel support*
   - *Heel cushions*
   - *Avoid flat shoes or going barefoot*

4. **Stretch your calves gently.** Reduces tension on the tendon. Stop if sharp pain occurs. Try:
   - *Wall calf stretch*
   - *Towel stretch (morning)*
   - *Standing calf stretch*

5. **Use MEAT after 48–72 hours**
   - **Movement:** Gentle ankle motion
   - **Exercise:** Strengthening, as tolerated
   - **Analgesics:** Pain relief if safe
   - **Treatment:** Massage or heat (after a few days)

6. **Switch to low-impact activity.** Until healing improves, try:
   - *Biking*
   - *Swimming*
   - *Elliptical machine*

Notes:

When to Seek Care

Right away if:

- You heard or felt a **"pop"**
- You can't **push off** the foot
- You can't **stand on your toes** (*These may be signs of a torn Achilles tendon*)

Within 1–2 weeks if:

- Pain isn't improving
- Swelling continues
- The tendon feels **thickened or lumpy**
- It hurts every time you try to be active
- Stiffness lasts more than 10–14 days
- Walking becomes harder

Your provider may recommend:

- Physical therapy
- Heel lifts
- Bracing or walking boot
- Imaging (ultrasound or MRI)
- Long-term issues may need special rehab or, in some cases, surgery

Key Terms

- **Achilles tendon:** The strong tendon that connects the calf muscles to the heel bone
- **Calf stretch:** A gentle stretch that loosens the calf muscles and reduces tension on the Achilles tendon
- **Heel lift:** A small pad placed in the shoe to reduce strain on the Achilles tendon
- **Tendonitis:** Irritation and inflammation of a tendon, usually causing pain and swelling
- **Tendinosis:** Long-term wear and tear of a tendon that leads to thickening and degeneration rather than swelling

Footnote Summary

- The Achilles tendon can become irritated from **overuse** or **tight calf muscles**
- **Pain, stiffness, and swelling** are common
- **Rest, ice, stretching, and supportive shoes** can help
- **Seek care** if pain lasts more than 1–2 weeks or if you heard a **"pop"**

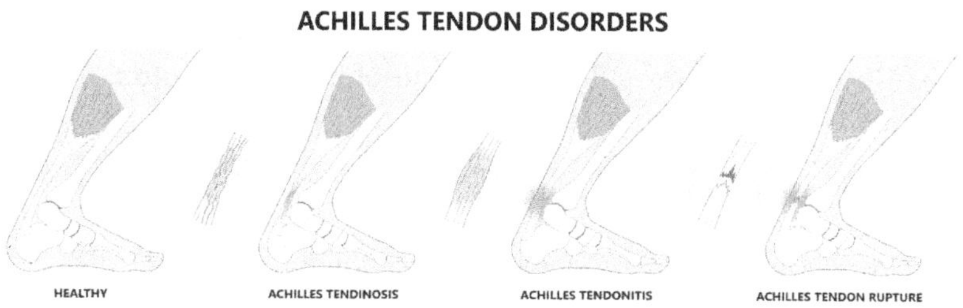

Achilles Tendon Rupture

What Is It?

An **Achilles tendon rupture** is a **tear** in the strong tendon that connects your **calf muscles to your heel**. It is a **medical emergency** that needs **prompt evaluation**. A rupture may be:

- **Partial:** Some tendon fibers tear
- **Complete:** The tendon splits entirely

Most people describe the injury as feeling like:

- A **sudden "pop"**
- A **sharp snap**
- Being **kicked in the back of the leg**
- Sudden pain that makes **walking very difficult**

Why It Happens

Ruptures often occur during movements involving **sudden force**, like jumping or sprinting.

Common causes include:

- Sudden push-off, sprinting, or jumping
- Falling or stepping into a hole
- **Tendonitis or tendinosis** that wasn't treated
- **Tight or weak calf muscles**
- Quick return to activity after rest
- **Middle age** (the tendon weakens over time)
- Certain medications (like **fluoroquinolones** or **steroids**) that increase tendon risk

What You Can Do at Home

If you think you have ruptured your Achilles tendon:

1. **Stop activity immediately.** Do *not* try to walk it off.

2. **Keep weight off the foot.** Use crutches or support from another person.

3. **Avoid stretching the tendon.** Stretching may worsen the tear.

4. **Apply ice.** 15–20 minutes at a time to reduce swelling.

5. **Elevate the foot.** Keep it gently raised to reduce swelling.

▲ A rupture **does not heal well on its own**. Most people will need a **boot, cast, or surgery**, depending on the tear.

This injury requires **urgent evaluation** by an **orthopedic** or **foot and ankle surgeon**.

When to Seek Care

Seek care immediately if you:

- Heard a **pop** in the back of your ankle
- **Cannot stand on your toes**
- **Cannot push off** the foot when walking
- Notice **swelling** or a "gap" where the tendon should be
- Are **limping** or unable to walk normally

What your provider may do:

- Physical exam
- Imaging (ultrasound or MRI)
- Discuss treatment options:
    - **Non-surgical** (boot or cast)
    - **Surgical repair**

Both options require **rest** and **physical therapy** to recover strength and flexibility.

Key Terms

- **Complete tear:** When the tendon is fully separated and no longer connected
- **Fluoroquinolone:** A type of antibiotic linked to tendon problems in some people
- **Partial tear:** When only some tendon fibers are torn, but some connection remains
- **Push-off:** The motion when your foot lifts the heel and steps forward
- **Rupture:** A significant tear in a tendon, often with sudden pain and loss of function

Footnote Summary

- An **Achilles rupture** is a serious tear in the tendon
- Often feels like a **"pop"** or being **kicked** in the leg
- You may not be able to **walk**, **push off**, or **stand on your toes**
- **Seek medical care immediately**—it requires **prompt treatment**

Notes:

Posterior Tibial Tendon Dysfunction (PTTD)

(Also called Adult-Acquired Flatfoot)

What Is It?

Posterior tibial tendon dysfunction (PTTD) occurs when the **posterior tibial tendon** becomes **weak, stretched, or torn**. This tendon runs along the **inside of the ankle** and helps support the **arch** of the foot.

When the tendon doesn't function properly, the **arch begins to collapse**, causing the foot to **roll inward**. This can lead to **pain, swelling, and difficulty walking**.

Common symptoms include:

- Pain along the **inside of the ankle**
- Swelling
- A **flattened arch**
- Trouble standing on your toes
- Foot that **rolls inward** when walking

Why It Happens

PTTD is a **progressive condition**, meaning it can worsen gradually over time. The tendon first becomes **strained**, then **stretched**, and may eventually **tear**.

Common causes include:

- Repeated ankle sprains
- Overuse (walking or standing all day)
- High-impact activity
- Tight or weak calf muscles
- Aging
- Flat feet
- Obesity
- Diabetes
- Inflammatory arthritis

What You Can Do at Home

1. **Avoid walking barefoot or wearing unsupportive shoes**
   Choose shoes with:
   - *Firm heel support*
   - *Arch support*
   - *Cushioning*

2. **Use orthotic inserts.** Arch supports reduce tendon strain. *Custom orthotics* may be helpful for persistent symptoms.

3. **Rest and support the tendon.** Reduce pain-causing activity. Use an *ankle brace or wrap* for added stability.

4. **Stretch the calf and foot.** Gentle stretching reduces tension on the tendon. Focus on:
   - *Calf stretches*
   - *Achilles stretches*

5. **Strengthen the tendon and arch.** Start slowly and increase as tolerated. Try:
   - *Heel raises*
   - *Short foot exercise*
   - *Towel scrunches*
   - *Resistance band exercises*

6. **Use RICE for soreness**
   At the end of the day or after activity:
   - **Rest**
   - **Ice**
   - **Compression**
   - **Elevation**

Notes:

When to Seek Care

Right away if you have:

- Sudden, sharp pain inside the ankle
- Inability to stand on your toes
- Worsening foot deformity
- Severe swelling

Within a few weeks if you notice:

- Pain not improving with home care
- Flattening of the arch
- Difficulty walking long distances
- Weakness or instability
- Uneven wear on shoes

⚠ **Early treatment helps prevent arch collapse.** Advanced cases may require **surgery** to repair or reconstruct the tendon and restore foot alignment.

Your provider may recommend:

- Physical therapy
- Custom orthotics
- Walking boot or brace
- Imaging (MRI or ultrasound)
- Anti-inflammatory medications or treatments

Key Terms

- **Adult-acquired flatfoot**: A type of arch collapse that develops over time, often due to tendon weakness
- **Dysfunction**: When something in the body is not working the way it should
- **Heel raise**: An exercise where you lift your heels off the ground to strengthen the calf and posterior tibial tendon
- **Orthotic**: A shoe insert designed to support the foot and improve alignment
- **Posterior tibial tendon**: The tendon on the inside of the ankle that supports the arch and helps with stability

Footnote Summary

- **PTTD** is caused by a **weakened tendon** on the inside of the ankle
- It can **flatten the arch** over time if untreated
- **Supportive shoes**, **orthotics**, and **strengthening exercises** are key
- **Seek care** if pain worsens or the arch keeps collapsing

Notes:

Peroneal Tendonitis / Peroneal Tendon Tears

What Is It?

The **peroneal tendons** are two tendons located on the **outside of your ankle**. They help **stabilize your foot** and **prevent ankle rolls**.

There are two peroneal tendons:

- **Peroneus longus**
- **Peroneus brevis**

Peroneal tendonitis means the tendons are **irritated and swollen**. **Peroneal tendon tears** can be **partial or complete**, and may require **MRI or ultrasound** to confirm.

Common symptoms include:

- Pain on the **outside of the ankle**
- Swelling
- Feeling like the ankle is **weak or unstable**
- Pain walking on uneven ground
- Pain **behind the ankle bone**
- Snapping feeling when the tendon moves

Why It Happens

According to AAOS, peroneal tendon problems often happen because the tendons must work hard to **keep the ankle steady**, especially **after sprains**. Tears may develop **slowly** from overuse or **suddenly** from a twisting injury.

Common causes include:

- Recent or repeated **ankle sprains**
- **High arches** (more pressure on peroneal tendons)
- Sudden increase in activity
- Walking or running on **uneven ground**
- Worn-out or unstable shoes
- Overuse from sports

What You Can Do at Home

1. **Rest and protect the ankle.** Avoid activities that increase pain on the outside of the ankle.

2. **Ice the area.** Apply for **15–20 minutes** a few times daily to reduce swelling.

3. **Use an ankle brace.** A supportive brace can **limit motion** and **protect the tendons**.

4. **Switch to safer activities.** Avoid running or hiking on rough surfaces. Try:
   - *Biking*
   - *Swimming*
   - *Elliptical*

5. **Wear supportive shoes.** Look for shoes with:
   - *Side-to-side stability*
   - *Firm heel support*
   - *Cushioning*

6. **Stretch and strengthen** (when pain improves)
   - *Calf stretches*
   - *Ankle circles*
   - *Resistance band exercises*
   - *Balance training*

7. **Use MEAT after 48–72 hours**
   - **Movement:** Gentle range-of-motion
   - **Exercise:** Light strengthening
   - **Analgesics:** Pain relievers if safe
   - **Treatment:** Heat or massage for stiffness

When to Seek Care

Right away if:

- You **cannot walk without limping**
- You heard a **"pop" on the outside** of the ankle
- The ankle looks **crooked or unstable**
- You have **numbness or tingling**

Within 1–2 weeks if:

- Pain **is not improving**
- Swelling keeps returning
- The ankle **keeps giving out**
- You feel **snapping, popping, or shifting**
- **Home care is not helping**

Your provider may recommend:

- Physical therapy
- Ankle brace or walking boot
- Custom orthotics
- Anti-inflammatory treatment
- Ultrasound or MRI

Severe or long-lasting tendon tears may require surgery to repair the tendon or stabilize the ankle.

Notes:

Tendonitis vs. Tendon Tear

Tendonitis	Tendon Tear
Pain develops over time	Often sudden pain after a specific event
Achy or burning pain	Sharp, intense pain
Swelling may be mild	Swelling and bruising more likely
Strength usually normal	Weakness is common
Walking is uncomfortable but possible	Walking may be very difficult
Usually improves with rest	Often needs medical evaluation or surgery

Decision Tree – Arch Pain

Does your arch look flatter than usual?
→ Yes → Go to next question
→ No → Could still be plantar fasciitis

Do you feel pain or swelling along the inside of your ankle?
→ Yes → Could be posterior tibial tendonitis
→ No → Go to next question

Does supportive footwear quickly improve symptoms?
→ Yes → Likely arch strain or early plantar fasciitis
→ No → Go to next question

Do you have burning or tingling?
→ Yes → Possible nerve irritation
→ No → Plantar fasciitis or overuse strain are likely

In Summary:

- ***Tendons*** *connect your muscles to bones and help you move and stay balanced.*
- *When tendons are* ***overused, irritated, or torn****, they can cause pain, swelling, and difficulty walking.*
- ***Most tendon problems improve*** *with a mix of* ***rest, stretching, strengthening, supportive footwear, and early care****.*
- *Avoid "pushing through" tendon pain—****listening to your body*** *helps prevent serious injury.*

Key Terms

- **Orthotic**: A shoe insert that improves support and helps keep the ankle in better alignment
- **Peroneal tendons**: The tendons on the outside of the ankle that help stabilize the foot and prevent it from rolling outward
- **Stability**: The ability of the ankle to stay steady and not "give out"
- **Tendon tear**: A rip in part or all of a tendon, which may cause weakness or pain
- **Tendonitis**: Irritation and swelling of a tendon, often caused by overuse or sudden increases in activity

Footnote Summary

- Peroneal tendon problems cause **pain on the outside of the ankle**
- They often happen after **sprains** or **overuse**
- **Rest, ice, bracing, and supportive shoes** help early healing
- **Seek care** if pain lasts more than 1–2 weeks or the ankle feels **unstable**

C. Fascia & Heel Disorders

Intro: Now let's look at the bottom of the foot, including the heel and plantar fascia. These tissues help absorb shock and support your arch, and they can become irritated from standing, walking, or wearing unsupportive shoes.

Plantar Fasciitis

What Is It?

Plantar fasciitis is one of the most common causes of **heel pain**. The **plantar fascia** is a thick band of tissue along the bottom of the foot. It connects the **heel to the toes** and supports your **foot arch**.

Plantar fasciitis occurs when this tissue becomes **inflamed, overstretched, or irritated**. Most people do **not recall a single injury**—symptoms tend to build **gradually over time**. The condition is **very common** and usually improves **without surgery**.

Common symptoms include:

- Sharp heel pain with the **first steps in the morning**
- Pain when standing after rest
- Discomfort in the **arch or bottom of the heel**
- **Tightness** in the calf muscles

Why It Happens

Plantar fasciitis is usually caused by **repeated strain** on the fascia.

Contributing factors include:

- Standing for long periods
- Walking or running on **hard surfaces**
- **Tight calf muscles**
- **Flat feet** or **high arches**
- Worn-out or unsupportive shoes
- Sudden increases in activity
- **Excess body weight**

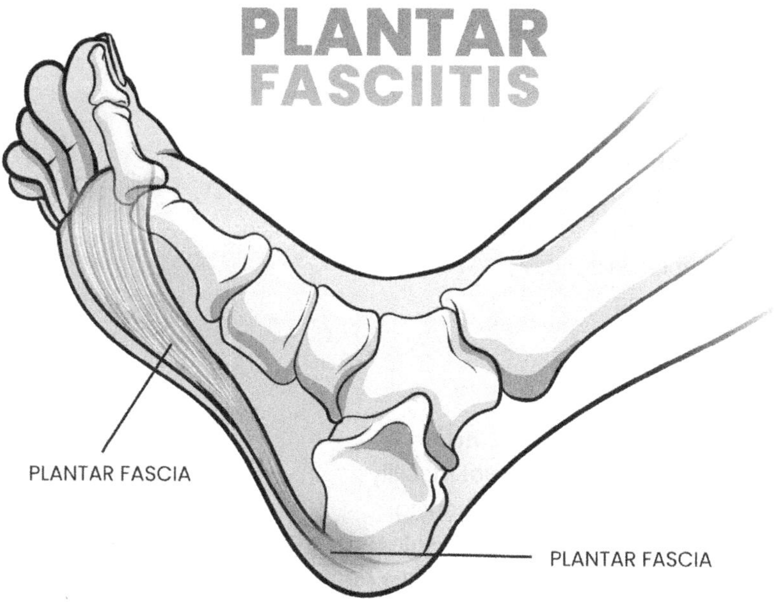

What You Can Do at Home

1. **Stretch your calves and plantar fascia.** Reduces tension and stress on the heel. Helpful stretches:
   • Wall calf stretch
   • Towel stretch before getting out of bed
   • Rolling your foot on a **cold water bottle**

2. **Ice the heel.** Apply ice or roll on a frozen water bottle for **15–20 minutes** to reduce inflammation.

3. **Wear supportive footwear.** Avoid **barefoot walking** and replace worn-out shoes. Look for:
   • Cushioned shoes
   • Shoes with **arch support**

4. **Use orthotic inserts.** Over-the-counter arch supports can reduce pressure on the heel. Custom orthotics may be recommended if pain persists.

5. **Try RICE for flare-ups**
    - **Rest**
    - **Ice**
    - **Compression** (if swollen)
    - **Elevation**

6. **Switch to low-impact activities** while healing
    Examples include:
    - Swimming
    - Biking
    - Elliptical

7. **Use MEAT after 48–72 hours**
    - **Movement:** Gentle foot mobility
    - **Exercise:** Foot strengthening
    - **Analgesics:** Pain relief if safe
    - **Treatment:** Massage or gentle heat

When to Seek Care

After 1–2 weeks if:

- Pain is not improving
- Morning pain remains intense
- Walking is becoming difficult
- You cannot return to regular activity

Right away if:

- You **cannot place weight** on the foot
- Sudden **heel swelling** occurs
- You experience **numbness or tingling**
- You feel a **"pop"** in the heel

These may suggest a more serious injury.

Your provider may recommend:

- Physical therapy
- Heel cups or **custom inserts**
- Night splints
- Anti-inflammatory treatment
- Imaging (ultrasound or MRI) if symptoms persist

Key Terms

- **Arch support:** A shoe or insert that supports the foot's natural arch
- **Inflammation:** Swelling and irritation of tissue
- **Low-impact exercise:** Activities that are gentle on the foot, such as swimming or cycling
- **Night splint:** A device worn during sleep to gently stretch the calf and foot
- **Plantar fascia:** A strong tissue band along the sole of the foot that supports the arch

Footnote Summary

- **Plantar fasciitis** is a common cause of **heel pain**
- Pain is often **worst in the morning** with first steps
- **Stretching, ice, and supportive shoes** help in most cases
- **Seek care** if symptoms last more than **1–2 weeks**

Notes:

Heel Pain (Including Heel Spurs)

What Is It?

Heel pain is one of the most common foot problems. Pain can be felt at the **bottom**, **back**, or **sides** of the heel depending on the cause.

A **heel spur** is a small bony growth on the bottom of the heel. These spurs often form in people with **plantar fasciitis** or long-term stress on the heel.

Heel spurs don't usually cause pain on their own. They are a sign of repeated stress on the heel—not the main problem.

Surgery for heel spurs is rarely needed, and only considered when all other treatments fail.

Common causes of heel pain include:

- **Plantar fasciitis** (most common)
- **Heel spurs**
- **Achilles tendonitis**
- **Bursitis**
- **Nerve irritation**

Typical symptoms:

- Sharp pain with **first steps in the morning**
- Pain after sitting or resting
- Tenderness or swelling
- Heel aching after long days
- Pain when wearing unsupportive shoes

Why It Happens

According to **AAOS** and **Mayo Clinic**, heel pain occurs when nearby tissues are **tight, irritated, or overworked**.

Common causes include:

- Plantar fasciitis
- Standing or walking all day
- Hard walking surfaces
- Worn-out or flat shoes
- High-impact activity
- Tight calf muscles
- Weight gain
- **Flat feet** or **high arches**
- **Fat pad thinning** (with age)
- Heel spur formation from stress

What You Can Do at Home

Stretch your calves and plantar fascia

- Wall calf stretches
- Towel stretch before getting out of bed
- Foot rolling on a tennis ball or frozen water bottle

Ice the heel. Apply ice for **15–20 minutes**, especially after activity.

Wear supportive shoes
Look for shoes with:

- Good arch support
- Cushioning
- Firm heel support
- Thick soles

🚫 Avoid:

- Flat shoes
- Flip-flops
- Thin soles
- Worn-out sneakers

Use orthotic inserts. Heel cups or store-bought inserts help cushion the heel and improve alignment.

Switch to low-impact exercise while healing

- Swimming
- Biking
- Elliptical

Use RICE for flare-ups

- **R**est
- **I**ce
- **C**ompression (if swollen)
- **E**levation

Use MEAT after early pain improves

- **M**ovement: gentle ankle range-of-motion
- **E**xercise: foot and calf strengthening
- **A**nalgesics: if safe for you
- **T**reatment: massage or heat

When to Seek Care

See a provider if:

- Pain lasts **more than 1–2 weeks**
- Morning pain is severe
- You can't walk comfortably
- Swelling doesn't improve
- Pain spreads into the **arch or toes**
- You have **numbness or tingling**
- You feel a **lump or bump** on the heel

Notes:

Your provider may recommend:

- Physical therapy
- Heel cups or **custom orthotics**
- Night splints
- Anti-inflammatory medications
- **Weight-bearing X-rays**
- **Ultrasound or MRI** for complex cases

Decision Tree: Heel Pain

Where is your pain worst?
→ First steps in the morning?
  → **Yes** → Likely **plantar fasciitis**
  → **No** → Go to next question

Does it improve after a few minutes of walking?
→ **Yes** → Likely **plantar fasciitis** or **arch strain**
→ **No** → Go to next question

Do you have numbness or tingling?
→ **Yes** → Possible **nerve issue** or **tarsal tunnel** — see provider
→ **No** → Go to next question

Is the pain sharp and at the bottom of the heel?
→ **Yes** → Classic **plantar fasciitis**
→ **No** → Consider **Achilles tendonitis** or **fat pad irritation**

Notes:

In Summary:

*Heel pain is very common because your heel absorbs the impact of every step. Problems usually build slowly but can flare from stress, shoes, or activity. Most heel pain improves with **stretching**, **supportive shoes**, and **home treatment**.*

▲ *Early care leads to faster recovery and helps avoid chronic issues.*

Key Terms

- **Bursitis:** Inflammation of a small fluid-filled sac that cushions joints and tendons
- **Heel spur:** A small bone growth on the bottom of the heel
- **Orthotic:** A supportive shoe insert that improves foot alignment
- **Plantar fascia:** Thick tissue on the bottom of the foot supporting the arch
- **Tendonitis:** Inflammation or irritation of a tendon

Footnote Summary

- Heel pain is usually from soft tissue irritation, **not** the bone spur
- **Supportive shoes, stretching, and ice** are effective first steps
- Seek care if pain **lasts more than 1–2 weeks** or impacts your daily life

Notes:

D. Joint & Bone Problems

Intro: Foot and ankle pain can also come from the joints and bones. These problems often develop slowly over time from wear-and-tear, arthritis, or changes in foot shape.

Arthritis (Ankle, Subtalar, Midfoot & Forefoot)

What Is It?

Arthritis can affect **any joint** in the foot or ankle, causing **pain**, **stiffness**, and **trouble walking**. With **33 joints** in the foot, arthritis is very common—especially after past injuries or with age.

This section covers arthritis in:
- The **ankle joint**
- The **subtalar joint** (below the ankle, side-to-side motion)
- The **midfoot** (middle arch area)
- The **forefoot** (toe joints, especially the big toe)

Arthritis happens when cartilage wears down, causing bones to rub together.

Common symptoms include:

- Deep aching joint pain
- Morning stiffness
- Swelling
- Pain with standing or walking
- "Start-up pain" after rest
- Difficulty walking on uneven ground (subtalar)
- Limited toe bending (forefoot)

Why It Happens

1. Previous injuries (most common cause):

- Old ankle sprains
- Past fractures
- Repeated joint trauma

2. Wear-and-tear (Osteoarthritis):

- Natural degeneration with time

3. Inflammatory arthritis:
Autoimmune conditions like:

- Rheumatoid arthritis
- Psoriatic arthritis
- Gout

4. Foot shape problems:

- Flat feet or high arches
- Bunions or toe deformities
- Joint misalignment placing stress on other joints

5. Aging:

- Cartilage thins and becomes less flexible with age

What You Can Do at Home

1. Wear supportive footwear. Choose shoes with:

- Stiff or **rocker-bottom soles**
- Soft cushioning
- Strong arch support
- Minimal toe bending

🚫 Avoid:

- Flexible, flimsy shoes
- Worn-out sneakers
- High heels

2. Use orthotic inserts. Helpful types include:

- Arch supports
- Carbon-fiber plates (to reduce toe joint bending)
- Heel cups
- Custom orthotics

3. Modify activity. Choose low-impact exercise:

- Swimming
- Biking
- Elliptical

🚫 Avoid:

- Running on hills
- High-impact sports
- Long walks on uneven terrain

4. Stretch and strengthen

- Stretch calves, hamstrings, and foot muscles
- Strengthen foot and ankle to reduce joint stress

5. Ice for swelling. Apply for 15–20 minutes after activity

6. Use MEAT when pain calms
Movement: gentle joint mobility
Exercise: strengthening and balance
Analgesics: pain relief (if safe for you)
Treatment: heat, massage, or joint support

7. Weight management. Even **small weight loss** reduces pressure on the ankle, midfoot, and big toe joints

When to Seek Care

See a foot & ankle specialist if:

- Pain lasts more than **1–2 weeks**
- Walking becomes difficult
- You feel **grinding or catching**
- Joint is stiff or visibly swollen
- Uneven ground worsens pain
- You can't bend your toes normally
- Home care stops helping

Your provider may recommend:

- X-rays to evaluate cartilage and alignment
- Physical therapy
- Custom orthotics or shoe modifications
- Anti-inflammatory medications
- Joint injections
- Bracing

Surgical options (if pain becomes severe):

- Joint cleaning (**debridement**)
- Bone spur removal
- **Joint fusion** (to stop painful motion)
- **Joint replacement** (mainly ankle or big toe)

Your surgeon will discuss options based on your **activity level** and **goals**.

Key Terms

- **Arthritis:** When joint cartilage wears down, causing pain and stiffness
- **Fusion:** Surgery that joins two bones to eliminate painful movement
- **Osteoarthritis:** Wear-and-tear arthritis that worsens with age or use
- **Rocker-bottom shoe:** A curved sole shoe that reduces the need for foot and ankle bending
- **Subtalar joint:** The joint below the ankle that controls side-to-side foot movement

Footnote Summary

- Arthritis can affect joints in the ankle, arch, or toes
- Symptoms include **pain**, **stiffness**, and **trouble walking**
- Supportive footwear, inserts, stretching, and modifying activities help
- Seek care if pain lasts more than **1–2 weeks** or limits function

Flat Foot

What Is It?

Flat feet—also called **fallen arches**—occur when the arch of the foot is **low or collapsed**. Some people are **born** with flat feet, while others **develop** them over time.

There are two main types:

- **Flexible Flat Feet (most common):** The arch appears flat **when standing**, but reappears **when sitting or lifting the foot**.

- **Rigid Flat Feet (less common):** The arch is **always flat** and the foot may feel **stiff** or limited in motion.

Flat feet in adults can cause:

- Arch pain
- Heel pain
- Achy or tired feet
- Swelling along the **inside of the ankle**
- Pain with standing or walking

Why It Happens

Adult flat feet often result from **posterior tibial tendon weakness**, which leads to **arch collapse**—called **adult-acquired flatfoot**.

Common causes include:

- Weak or overstretched **posterior tibial tendon**
- Repeated ankle sprains or stress
- **Aging**
- **Obesity**
- **Arthritis** or **diabetes**
- **Tight Achilles tendon**

What You Can Do at Home

1. Wear supportive shoes. Look for shoes with:

- Strong **arch support**
- **Firm heel counter**
- Soft **cushioning**

🚫 Avoid:

- Flip-flops
- Worn-out shoes
- Flat shoes with no support

2. Use orthotic inserts

- **Over-the-counter arch supports** help many people
- **Custom orthotics** may be needed if pain continues

3. Stretch the calves and Achilles tendon. Tight calf muscles can worsen flat foot symptoms. Try:

- Wall calf stretch
- Towel stretch (especially in the morning)
- Ankle mobility exercises

4. Strengthen the arch and foot muscles. Try these simple exercises:

- Towel scrunches
- Marble pickups
- Toe spreading
- "Short foot" exercise (gently lift the arch)

5. Use RICE for soreness. If feet ache after long days:
Rest, **Ice**, **Compression**, **Elevation**

6. Maintain a healthy weight. Extra weight puts additional pressure on arches and tendons

When to Seek Care

See a foot and ankle specialist if you experience:

- Pain along the **inside of the ankle**
- Arch or heel pain that doesn't improve
- Ongoing **swelling**
- Difficulty standing for long periods
- A foot that keeps **rolling inward**
- **Progressive flattening** of the foot

Your provider may recommend:

- Physical therapy
- Custom orthotics
- Ankle **bracing**
- Imaging (X-ray, ultrasound, or MRI)
- Treatment for **posterior tibial tendon dysfunction**
- In severe cases: **surgical correction**

Key Terms

- **Adult-acquired flatfoot:** Arch collapse that develops later in life, often due to tendon failure
- **Arch:** The curved part of the foot that helps absorb shock and support body weight
- **Flexible flat foot:** A flat arch that returns when the foot is not bearing weight
- **Posterior tibial tendon:** A tendon along the inner ankle that helps support the arch
- **Rigid flat foot:** A flat arch that stays flat even when off the ground

Footnote Summary

- Flat feet are common and often painless—especially in children.
- In adults, they can cause pain or fatigue due to **tendon weakness**.
- **Supportive shoes**, **stretching**, and **strengthening** exercises help.
- Seek care if pain, swelling, or progressive flattening develops.

Notes:

Hallux Rigidus (Big Toe Arthritis)

What Is It?

Hallux rigidus is arthritis of the **big toe joint**—where your big toe meets your foot. Because this joint bends with every step, arthritis here can make **daily walking painful**. The word **rigidus** means "**stiff big toe**."

This is similar to "wear-and-tear" arthritis in a **knee or hip**, but it affects the big toe. As cartilage wears down, bones rub together, causing **pain, stiffness,** and **bone spurs**.

Common symptoms include:

- Pain in the big toe joint
- Stiffness, especially in the morning
- Swelling or tenderness
- Trouble bending the toe upward
- Pain when pushing off the foot
- A bump on top of the big toe joint (bone spur)

Why It Happens

According to **AAOS** and **Johns Hopkins**, hallux rigidus occurs when the **cartilage in the big toe joint wears down over time.**

Common causes include:

- Overuse or repeated stress
- Prior injury (e.g. turf toe, sprains)
- High-impact sports
- Genetics (runs in families)
- Flat feet or poor foot alignment
- Arthritis conditions

Notes:

What You Can Do at Home

1. Wear stiff-soled or rocker-bottom shoes. These reduce bending of the big toe and relieve pain.

Good options:

- Thick-soled shoes
- Hiking or walking shoes
- Rocker-bottom shoes

🚫 Avoid:

- Flexible shoes
- High heels
- Tight shoes

2. Ice and elevation. Apply ice for **15–20 minutes** after activity to calm swelling.

3. Use anti-inflammatory medication *(if safe for you).* This helps reduce swelling and pain. Ask your provider before using NSAIDs.

4. Try orthotic inserts or carbon-fiber plates. These limit painful toe motion and support the joint.

5. Modify your activity. Avoid painful movements like running hills or pushing off forcefully. Try:

- Biking
- Swimming
- Rowing

6. Gentle stretching. Stretch the **calf** and **bottom of the foot** to reduce pressure on the big toe joint.

Notes:

When to Seek Care

See a specialist if:

- Pain lasts more than 1–2 weeks
- The big toe becomes stiff or hard to bend
- Walking is painful or difficult
- A bump is forming over the joint
- Home care isn't helping
- Pain interferes with daily life

Your provider may recommend:

- **X-rays** to check joint space and bone spurs
- **Custom orthotics** or **stiff-soled shoes**
- **Physical therapy**
- **Anti-inflammatory treatment**
- **Steroid injections** (in selected cases)

If arthritis is severe, surgery may be needed, such as:

- Bone spur removal
- Joint cleaning (**cheilectomy**)
- **Fusion surgery** (most common)
- **Joint replacement** (less common)

Your surgeon will help decide which option fits your **pain level**, **joint motion**, and **activity needs**.

In Summary:
*Joint and bone issues in the foot often develop **gradually** due to aging, activity, or old injuries. While arthritis can't always be reversed, many people feel better with the **right shoes, therapy, and activity changes**. The focus is on **pain relief and keeping you moving**.*

Notes:

Key Terms

- **Arthritis**: Wear-and-tear damage to a joint that causes pain and stiffness
- **Bone spur**: Extra bone that forms due to irritation or stress in a joint
- **Cheilectomy**: Surgery that removes bone spurs from the big toe joint to improve motion
- **Hallux**: The medical term for the big toe
- **Rigidus**: Means "stiff"; refers to limited big toe movement

Footnote Summary

- Hallux rigidus is **arthritis of the big toe joint**
- It causes **pain, stiffness**, and **difficulty walking or pushing off**
- **Supportive shoes**, **inserts**, and **activity changes** are helpful
- Seek care if pain **lasts over 1–2 weeks** or interferes with daily activity

Notes:

E. Forefoot Mechanics & Toe Deformities

Intro: The front of the foot, called the forefoot, includes the toes and the ball of the foot. This area handles a lot of pressure when you walk, and problems here can cause pain with standing, shoes, or activity.

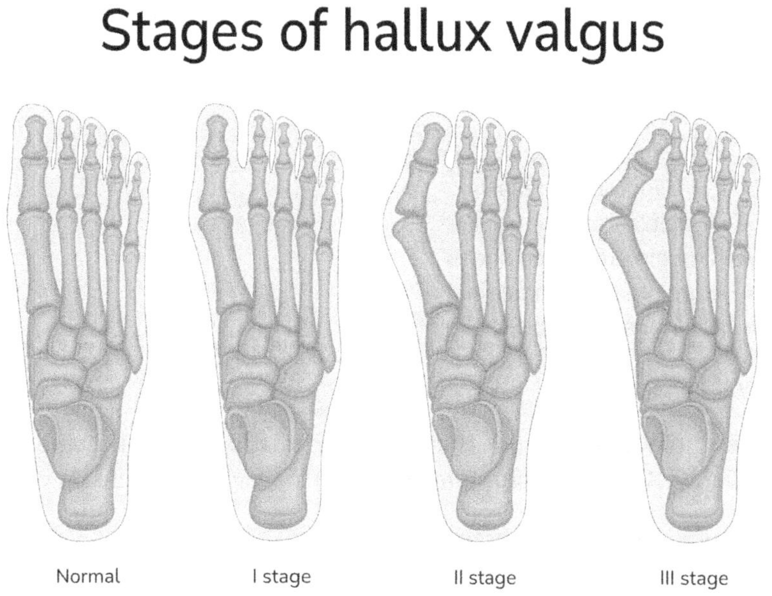

Notes:

Bunion (Hallux Valgus)

What Is It?

A **bunion** is a bony bump that forms at the **base of the big toe**, where the toe meets the foot.

As the bump grows, the **big toe begins to lean toward the second toe**, leading to pain, pressure, and trouble finding comfortable shoes.

A bunion isn't just a surface bump — it's a **misalignment of bones** in the front of the foot.

Symptoms may include:

- Pain on the inner side of the big toe
- Swelling or redness
- A visible bump
- Trouble fitting into shoes
- Burning or aching pain
- Stiffness in the big toe joint

Why It Happens

Bunions form when the bones in the front of the foot slowly become misaligned. Over time, pressure on the big toe joint pushes it sideways.

Common contributing factors:

- Tight, narrow, or pointed shoes
- High heels
- Flat feet or unstable arches
- Family history of bunions
- Loose ligaments or flexible joints
- Arthritis (especially **rheumatoid arthritis**)
- Previous foot injuries

What You Can Do at Home

1. Wear wider shoes. Choose footwear with:

- A **wide toe box**
- **Good arch support**
- **Low or no heel**

🚫 Avoid shoes that squeeze your toes together.

2. Use bunion pads or cushions. These help reduce rubbing and pressure on the bump.

3. Ice the area. Apply ice for **15–20 minutes** after long days to reduce pain and swelling.

4. Try toe spacers. Soft spacers between the toes can help keep the big toe straighter and reduce rubbing.

5. Strengthen and stretch. These can reduce strain on the joint. Try:

- Towel scrunches
- Toe spreading
- Big toe flexion and extension
- Calf stretches

6. Use orthotic inserts. Over-the-counter arch supports may help relieve pressure and slow progression.

7. Modify your activity. Avoid long walks in tight shoes or high-impact activity during flare-ups.

Notes:

When to Seek Care

See a specialist if:

- Pain doesn't improve with wider shoes
- The bump keeps getting larger
- Walking becomes difficult
- You can't straighten your big toe
- Your second toe begins to overlap the first
- You have burning, tingling, or numbness

Your provider may recommend:

- Custom orthotics
- Physical therapy
- Padding or taping
- Anti-inflammatory treatment
- Night splints
- Weight-bearing X-rays to check alignment

If pain is **severe** or interfering with daily life, **surgery may be an option** to correct the bone alignment. Surgery is **not always necessary**, and many people find relief with conservative treatment.

Key Terms

- **Alignment**: How the bones of the foot line up when standing or walking
- **Bunion**: A bony bump at the base of the big toe due to bone misalignment
- **Orthotic**: A shoe insert that supports the foot and improves alignment
- **Toe box**: The front part of a shoe that houses the toes; wider shapes reduce pressure
- **Toe spacer**: A soft insert placed between toes to reduce rubbing and shift alignment

Footnote Summary

- A bunion is a **bony bump caused by bone misalignment**
- **Tight or narrow shoes** can make it worse
- Try **wide shoes**, **pads**, **ice**, and **inserts**
- Seek care if the **bunion grows** or **walking becomes painful**

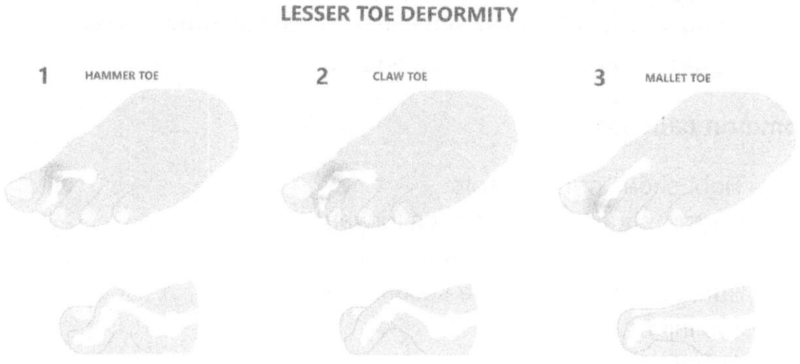

Hammertoe

What Is It?

A **hammertoe** is a toe that stays bent at the middle joint, giving it a curled or "hammer-like" appearance. It most often affects the **second toe**, but can occur in any toe.

There are two main types:

- **Flexible hammertoe**: The toe can still move or straighten
- **Rigid hammertoe**: The toe is stiff and stuck in a bent position

Symptoms may include:

- A toe that bends downward
- Pain or rubbing on the **top of the toe**
- Corns or calluses
- Trouble fitting into shoes
- Tenderness where shoes press on the toe

Why It Happens

Hammertoes develop when the **muscles and tendons** controlling the toe become imbalanced. This imbalance gradually **pulls the toe into a bent position**, which may become permanent over time.

Common causes:

- Tight shoes or high heels
- Narrow shoes that push toes forward
- Family history of foot deformities
- Bunions (which push the second toe upward)
- Toe injury
- Arthritis
- High arches (increase pressure on toes)
- Weak foot muscles

What You Can Do at Home

1. Wear wider, deeper shoes. Look for:

- A **wide toe box**
- Soft or stretchy materials
- **Low heels**

🚫 Avoid tight or pointed shoes.

2. Use toe pads or cushions. These can reduce rubbing and pressure on the top of the bent toe.

3. Try toe spacers. Helps align the toe and minimize friction between toes.

4. Strengthen and stretch the toes. Especially helpful for **flexible hammertoes**. Try:

- Towel scrunches
- Marble pickups
- Toe extension and flexion
- Gently pulling the toe into a straight position

5. Use orthotic inserts. These help improve foot alignment and reduce pressure on the toes, especially if you also have a **bunion** or **flatfoot**.

6. Ice for pain or swelling. Apply ice for **15–20 minutes** after activity or irritation.

When to Seek Care

See a provider if:

- The toe becomes **stiff** and hard to straighten
- Pain is **getting worse**
- Shoes are hard to wear comfortably
- Corns or calluses keep coming back
- The toe overlaps or pushes into another toe
- You also have a **bunion** that worsens the deformity

If the hammertoe becomes rigid or painful, **surgery** may be considered to straighten the toe or release tight tissues.

Your provider may recommend:

- Custom orthotics
- Shoe modifications
- Splints or taping
- Physical therapy
- Anti-inflammatory treatment
- X-rays to check joint and alignment

Key Terms

- **Callus**: Thickened skin that forms from pressure or friction, often on top of bent toes
- **Flexibility**: How easily a joint moves or straightens
- **Hammertoe**: A deformity where the toe bends downward at the middle joint
- **Orthotic**: A shoe insert that improves foot alignment and reduces toe pressure
- **Toe box**: The front part of a shoe where the toes sit; wider boxes reduce toe irritation

Footnote Summary

- A hammertoe is a **toe bent at the middle joint**
- Caused by **muscle imbalance**, **tight shoes**, or **bunion pressure**
- **Wide shoes**, **toe exercises**, and **pads** help in early stages
- Seek care if the toe becomes **stiff**, **painful**, or **hard to fit into shoes**

Notes:

Metatarsalgia *(Pain in the Ball of the Foot)*

What Is It?

Metatarsalgia is a common condition that causes **pain in the ball of the foot** — the area just behind the toes. This pain usually **builds gradually** and often feels like burning, sharp discomfort, or pressure.

People often describe:

- "Walking on a pebble"
- Pain that worsens with activity
- Soreness when standing for long periods
- Burning or aching in the front of the foot
- Pain that improves with rest

Metatarsalgia is a **symptom**, not a disease. It happens when the front of the foot is under **too much stress**.

Why It Happens

Metatarsalgia develops when there is **extra pressure on the metatarsal bones** (the long bones behind your toes).

Common causes include:

- High-impact sports
- Long-distance walking or running
- Tight or thin-soled shoes
- High heels
- Foot deformities (bunions, hammertoes)
- Flat feet or high arches
- Excess body weight
- Standing for long periods
- Loss of fat padding in the foot (common with aging)

Anything that increases pressure on the **ball of the foot** can lead to pain.

What You Can Do at Home

1. Wear supportive footwear. Choose shoes that:

- Have good **cushioning** under the ball of the foot
- Provide **arch support**
- Include a **wide toe box**

🚫 Avoid:

- High heels
- Thin-soled shoes
- Tight shoes

2. Use metatarsal pads. These soft pads are placed **just behind the painful area** to reduce pressure.

3. Apply ice after activity. Ice for **15–20 minutes** to calm irritation.

4. Rest or modify activity. Temporarily switch to **low-impact exercise** and reduce:

- Running
- Jumping
- Long walks on hard surfaces

5. Stretch tight muscles. Stretching the **calf** and **bottom of the foot** can reduce forefoot stress.

6. Use orthotic inserts. Over-the-counter or **custom orthotics** can help with cushioning and realignment.

7. Try MEAT as pain improves

- **Movement**: gentle foot mobility
- **Exercise**: gradual strengthening
- **Analgesics**: for pain relief (if safe)
- **Treatment**: warm compresses or massage

When to Seek Care

You should see a provider if:

- Pain lasts **more than 1–2 weeks**
- Pain **interferes with walking or activity**
- Swelling does not improve
- Pain **returns after each activity**
- You have **bunion or toe deformities** adding pressure
- You suspect a **stress fracture**

Your provider may recommend:

- Physical therapy
- Custom orthotics
- Shoe modifications
- Padding
- X-rays to check bone alignment or rule out fractures
- MRI if symptoms persist

Key Terms

- **Cushioning**: Padding that absorbs impact and reduces pressure on the foot
- **Metatarsal pad**: A small insert placed behind the ball of the foot to ease pressure
- **Metatarsals**: Long bones in the forefoot just behind the toes
- **Metatarsalgia**: Pain in the ball of the foot caused by stress on the metatarsals
- **Orthotic**: A shoe insert that improves foot alignment and reduces pressure points

Footnote Summary

- Metatarsalgia = **pain in the ball of the foot** from pressure or overuse
- Supportive shoes, pads, stretching, and rest can help
- Seek care if pain **lasts more than 1–2 weeks** or **keeps returning**

Sesamoiditis

What Is It?

Sesamoiditis is irritation or inflammation of the **sesamoid bones**—two tiny bones under the big toe joint. These bones act like pulleys, helping your big toe move and absorb pressure during walking and running.

When the **tendons around the sesamoids** become irritated, you may feel:

- Pain under the big toe joint
- Tenderness when pushing off
- Swelling or warmth
- Pain in thin or flexible shoes
- Pain that worsens with running or jumping

Why It Happens

Sesamoiditis develops when the **front of the foot is under repetitive stress**, especially during high-impact or toe-off movements.

Common causes include:

- Running or dancing
- Jumping sports
- High heels or thin-soled shoes
- Sudden increase in activity
- High arches (increase pressure on sesamoids)

- Foot shape that puts extra weight on the big toe
- Tight calf muscles
- Repetitive stress

SESAMOIDITIS

RESULTS FROM OVERUSE OF THE TENDONS SURROUNDING THE SESAMOID BONES SUCH AS WEARING HIGH HEELS OR SPORTS ACTIVITIES CAN LEAD TO IRRITATED AND INFLAMED

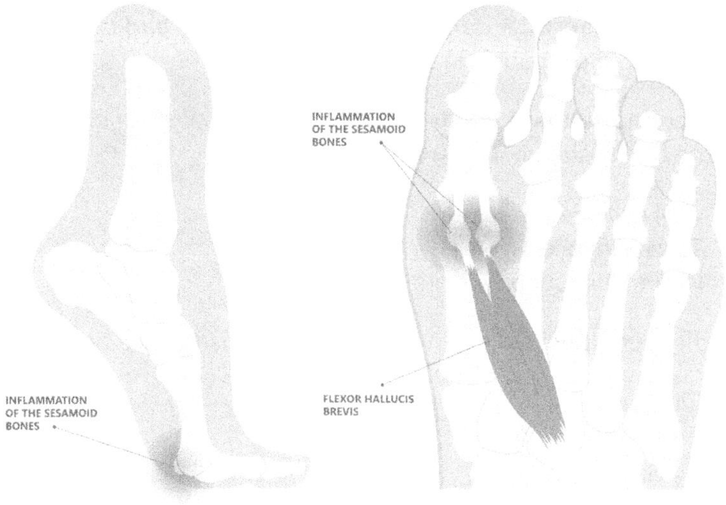

☛ It can also occur after a **sesamoid stress fracture**, which may need imaging to diagnose.

What You Can Do at Home

1. Rest the foot. Limit or avoid activities that worsen the pain—especially high-impact ones.

2. Ice the painful area. Use ice for **15–20 minutes**, especially after walking or exercise.

3. Wear cushioned or stiff-soled shoes. Choose shoes with:

- Thick soles
- Good forefoot cushioning
- A firm bottom (rocker-bottom shoes can help)

🚫 Avoid:

- High heels
- Very flexible shoes
- Barefoot walking

4. Use pad supports. A **dancer's pad** or **sesamoid pad** can offload pressure from the big toe joint.

5. Stretch the calf and plantar fascia. Tight muscles can increase pressure on the sesamoids. Try:

- Wall calf stretch
- Towel stretches
- Rolling the foot on a ball

6. Modify activities. Switch to low-impact exercises while healing:

- Biking
- Swimming
- Elliptical

7. Try MEAT once pain calms down

- **Movement**: gentle foot motion
- **Exercise**: as tolerated
- **Analgesics**: pain relievers if safe
- **Treatment**: warm compress or gentle massage

When to Seek Care

You should see a provider if:

- Pain lasts **more than 1–2 weeks**
- It's painful to **walk or push off**
- Swelling does not go down
- You feel **sharp pain under the big toe**
- You suspect a **stress fracture**
- Pain returns every time activity increases

Your provider may recommend:

- **X-rays** (first step)
- **MRI or ultrasound** if pain persists
- **Custom orthotics**
- **Stiff-soled shoes** or a **walking boot**
- **Physical therapy**
- **Anti-inflammatory treatment**

In cases of severe irritation or fracture, temporary immobilization in a boot may be needed.

Key Terms

- **Sesamoid bones**: Two small bones under the big toe joint
- **Inflammation**: Swelling and irritation in tissue
- **Dancer's pad**: A pad placed behind the big toe joint to reduce pressure
- **Rocker-bottom shoe**: A shoe with a curved sole that eases forefoot stress
- **Stress fracture**: A small crack in a bone caused by overuse or pressure

Footnote Summary

- Sesamoiditis = **inflammation of tiny bones** under the big toe
- Pain is common when **pushing off** or wearing thin shoes
- Rest, pads, ice, and supportive shoes can help
- Seek care if pain lasts over 1–2 weeks or makes walking difficult

Notes:

In Summary

*The **forefoot handles a lot of pressure** during push-off and standing, which is why problems here are so common. Pain may come from the **joints, tendons, bones**, or even small changes in **toe alignment**.*

Many forefoot issues respond well to:

- *Shoe changes*
- *Padding*
- *Stretching*
- *Avoiding tight or unsupportive footwear*

If pain affects walking, causes swelling, or keeps coming back, an evaluation can help find the best treatment.

Notes:

F. Nerve Problems

Intro: Some foot and ankle pain comes from the nerves. Nerve problems can cause burning, tingling, numbness, or sharp shooting pain. These conditions often feel very different from joint or tendon pain.

Tarsal Tunnel Syndrome

What is it?

Tarsal tunnel syndrome happens when the **tibial nerve** gets pinched or compressed as it travels through a tight space called the **tarsal tunnel**, located on the inside of the ankle. Think of it like **"carpal tunnel syndrome"**—but in the foot.

Symptoms often come and go at first and may worsen over time.

You may feel:

- Burning or tingling on the inside of the ankle
- Numbness or shooting pain into the arch, heel, or toes
- A "pins and needles" feeling
- Pain that worsens with standing or walking
- Foot fatigue or weakness

Why it happens

According to AAOS and Johns Hopkins, anything that puts pressure on the tibial nerve inside the tunnel can cause tarsal tunnel syndrome.

Common causes include:

- Flat feet (arch collapse stretches the nerve)
- Swelling from an ankle injury
- Varicose veins near the nerve
- Bone spurs
- Cysts or masses (rare)
- Tight shoes or ankle braces
- Arthritis
- Diabetes (increases nerve sensitivity)
- Overuse or long periods of standing

Sometimes the exact cause is unclear—nerve irritation may build slowly over time.

What you can do at home

1. Rest and reduce irritating activity. Avoid long walks or standing for long periods.

2. Ice the inside of the ankle. Ice for 15–20 minutes to reduce swelling around the nerve.

3. Wear supportive shoes. Avoid tight shoes or stiff ankle braces. Choose shoes that:

- Support the arch
- Have good cushioning
- Do not press against the inside of the ankle

4. Use orthotic inserts. Arch supports reduce nerve pressure, especially helpful with flat feet.

5. Stretch the calf and foot
Gentle stretching improves alignment and reduces nerve tension.

6. Try MEAT when symptoms calm

- **M**ovement: gentle ankle mobility
- **E**xercise: foot and ankle strengthening
- **A**nalgesics: pain relief if safe
- **T**reatment: massage or warm compresses

7. Modify activities. Choose low-impact options until symptoms improve:

- Swimming
- Biking
- Elliptical

When to seek care

See a specialist if:

- Pain lasts more than 1–2 weeks
- You have numbness or tingling in the sole of the foot
- Sharp, burning pain spreads into the toes
- You feel weakness or foot fatigue
- Home care is not helping
- Symptoms worsen with activity

Your provider may recommend:

- Physical therapy
- Custom orthotics
- Anti-inflammatory medication
- Nerve gliding exercises
- Ultrasound or MRI
- Steroid injections (in some cases)

If symptoms are **severe** or do not improve, **surgery** may be considered to release pressure on the nerve.

Key Terms

- **Tibial nerve**: Nerve that travels behind the inside ankle
- **Compression**: Pressure on a nerve
- **Arch support**: Insert that helps align the foot
- **Numbness**: Reduced or absent feeling
- **Tarsal tunnel**: Narrow space where the tibial nerve runs

Footnote Summary

- Tarsal tunnel syndrome is **nerve irritation** on the inside of the ankle.
- Symptoms include **burning, tingling, numbness**, and pain with standing.
- **Supportive shoes, stretching, and rest** often help.
- Seek care if symptoms last more than 1–2 weeks or worsen with activity.

Morton's Neuroma

What is it?

A **Morton's neuroma** is a painful swelling or irritation of a **nerve in the ball of the foot**.

It usually forms between the **third and fourth toes**, but can occur between other toes.

It is **not a tumor**, despite the name. It is a **thickened, irritated nerve** caused by compression or repeated stress.

Common symptoms include:

- Sharp or burning pain in the ball of the foot
- A feeling like a "pebble in your shoe"
- Tingling or numbness in the toes
- Pain that gets worse in tight shoes

Why it happens

Morton's neuroma occurs when a **nerve becomes pinched between the metatarsal bones**. Over time, pressure on the nerve causes it to thicken and become painful.

Common causes include:

- Tight or narrow shoes
- High heels
- Shoes with a tight toe box
- Repetitive stress on the forefoot
- Running or high-impact sports
- Flat feet or high arches
- Toe deformities (such as bunions or hammertoes)

Notes:

What you can do at home

1. Change your footwear. Avoid shoes that squeeze the toes. Choose shoes that:

- Have a **wide toe box**
- Provide **cushioning** in the ball of the foot
- Have a **low or no heel**

Avoid:

- High heels
- Pointy or tight shoes
- Narrow athletic shoes

2. Use metatarsal pads or inserts. These soft pads sit behind the ball of the foot to offload pressure from the nerve.

3. Rest from high-impact activities. Avoid running, jumping, or anything that irritates the forefoot. Good alternatives include:

- Swimming
- Biking
- Elliptical

4. Ice the painful area. Apply ice for **15–20 minutes** after activity to calm inflammation.

5. Massage the foot. Gentle massage can help loosen tight tissues around the nerve.

6. Try MEAT when pain calms down

- **Movement:** gentle foot mobility
- **Exercise:** calf and foot strengthening
- **Analgesics:** pain relief if safe for you
- **Treatment:** warm compresses or stretching

When to seek care

See a specialist if:

- Pain lasts more than 2 weeks
- You feel numbness or tingling in the toes
- Shoe changes and pads don't help
- Pain keeps returning or limits activity
- You feel like your sock is "bunched up" under your foot

Your provider may recommend:

- Custom orthotics
- Physical therapy
- Padding or shoe modifications
- Anti-inflammatory treatment
- Ultrasound or MRI if symptoms persist
- Injections or, in rare cases, surgery to relieve nerve pressure

Key Terms

- **Ball of the foot**: The area just behind the toes that takes pressure when you walk
- **Compression**: Pressure or squeezing on a nerve that can cause pain, tingling, or numbness
- **Metatarsal pads**: Soft pads placed behind the ball of the foot to reduce pressure on the nerve
- **Neuroma**: A thickened, irritated nerve that can cause burning, numbness, or sharp pain in the toes
- **Toe box**: The front part of a shoe where the toes sit; a wider toe box can reduce nerve irritation

Notes:

Footnote Summary

- Morton's neuroma is a **swollen nerve** in the ball of the foot
- Tight shoes and high heels are common causes
- Wide shoes, padding, and ice can help
- Seek care if pain lasts more than **2 weeks** or you feel numbness

Lumbar Radiculopathy (Foot & Ankle Pain From the Spine)

What is it?

Lumbar radiculopathy means a **nerve** in the lower back is irritated or pinched. Even though the problem starts in the spine, the pain can travel down the leg into the:

- Foot
- Ankle
- Heel
- Toes

You may feel:

- Sharp or shooting pain in the foot
- Numbness or tingling
- Burning or electric-like pain
- Weakness in the foot or toes
- Pain that worsens with sitting or bending
- Relief when lying down or changing position

Why it happens

According to AAOS and Mayo Clinic, lumbar radiculopathy occurs when something compresses a spinal nerve in the lower back.

Notes:

Common causes include:

- Herniated disc
- Arthritis of the spine
- Bone spurs
- Spinal stenosis (narrowing of the canal)
- Muscle tightness or spasms
- Age-related wear-and-tear

The part of the foot affected depends on which nerve is involved:

- **L4 nerve:** inner foot and ankle
- **L5 nerve:** top of the foot or big toe
- **S1 nerve:** outside of the foot or sole

What you can do at home

1. Change positions frequently. Gentle movement helps calm irritated nerves.Avoid long periods of:

- Sitting
- Standing
- Bending forward

2. Use ice or heat. Use for 15–20 minutes at a time.

- Ice for sharp or recent pain
- Heat for tight muscles or stiffness

3. Stretch key muscle groups. Tight muscles can increase nerve pressure. Gently stretch:

- Hamstrings
- Hips
- Low back

4. Take short walks. Walking is one of the best activities for mild radiculopathy.

5. Avoid heavy lifting. Especially lifting with your back bent forward.

6. Try over-the-counter medicines (if safe). NSAIDs or acetaminophen may help reduce pain.

7. Wear supportive shoes. Good footwear reduces leg strain and may ease nerve symptoms in the foot.

When to seek care

See a specialist if:

- Pain lasts more than 1–2 weeks
- Symptoms keep traveling down the leg
- You have numbness in the foot or toes
- You feel weakness when lifting the foot
- Pain worsens despite home care
- Walking becomes difficult

Seek emergency care if:

- You **lose control** of your bladder or bowel
- You have **sudden**, severe weakness
- You cannot walk normally

These may be signs of serious nerve compression.

Your provider may recommend:

- Physical therapy
- Medication for nerve pain
- Imaging (MRI if needed)
- Steroid injections
- A referral to a spine specialist

Most cases **do not** require surgery, and many improve with conservative care.

Key Terms

- **Herniated disc:** When the soft inner part of a spinal disc pushes out and presses on a nerve
- **Nerve root:** The start of a nerve where it exits the spine
- **Radiculopathy:** A pinched spinal nerve causing pain, numbness, or weakness
- **Sciatica:** A general term for nerve pain radiating down the leg
- **Stenosis:** Narrowing of the spinal canal that can put pressure on nerves

Footnote Summary

- Lumbar radiculopathy is **nerve irritation** in the lower back that can cause foot or ankle pain
- Symptoms may include burning, tingling, or **shooting** pain
- Stretching, walking, and posture changes often help
- Seek care if pain lasts more than 1–2 weeks or causes weakness

In Summary

- *Nerve-related foot and ankle pain often feels very different from joint, tendon, or bone problems. It may cause **burning, tingling, numbness**, or **electric-shock sensations**.*
- *While the pain might be felt in the foot, the source can be higher up—such as the **ankle, midfoot, or even the lower back**.*
- *Early diagnosis is important because nerve conditions respond best to the **right combination of stretching, supportive footwear, activity changes, medications, or injections**.*
- *Left untreated, nerve pain can become harder to manage over time.*

G. Skin & Nail Disorders

The skin and nails of the feet can also cause discomfort, especially when irritated, infected, or difficult to trim. These conditions are common and often easy to treat with the right care.

Ingrown Toenails

What are they?

An **ingrown toenail** happens when the edge of a toenail grows into the skin next to it. This most often affects the big toe.

In early stages, it may be only mildly sore. If the nail keeps digging in, the skin can become very irritated or even infected.

You may notice:

- Redness
- Swelling
- Tenderness
- Pain when wearing shoes
- Drainage or signs of infection (in more severe cases)

Why it happens

According to **Cleveland Clinic** and **Mayo Clinic**, ingrown toenails are usually caused by **pressure**, **improper nail trimming**, or **toe injuries**.
Some people naturally have nails that curve more, which increases the risk.

Common causes include:

- Cutting toenails too short
- Rounding the edges instead of cutting straight across
- Tight shoes or narrow toe boxes
- Toe trauma (stubbing the toe or dropping something on it)
- Thick or curved nails
- Sweaty feet (softens the skin)
- Poor foot hygiene

What you can do at home

1. Soak the foot in warm water. Do this for 15–20 minutes to soften the skin and reduce tenderness.. Do this 2–3 times a day.

2. Wear roomy shoes. Avoid tight shoes that press on the big toe. Choose shoes with:

- A wide toe box
- Breathable material
- Low heels

3. Keep the toe clean and dry. Dry the area fully after bathing. This helps prevent moisture buildup and skin breakdown.

4. Gently lift the nail edge (ONLY if mild). After soaking, you may try placing a small piece of **cotton or dental floss** under the nail to reduce pressure.

Stop if this causes pain or bleeding.

5. Over-the-counter pain relief. Short-term use of acetaminophen or NSAIDs may reduce pain and swelling.

6. Avoid cutting into the nail edge. Cutting the nail deeper often worsens the problem and increases the risk of infection.

7. Do not pick or peel at the nail. Picking can break the skin and allow bacteria to enter.

When to seek care

See a specialist if:

- Pain becomes severe
- Redness or swelling spreads
- You see drainage or pus
- The skin begins to grow over the nail
- Home care doesn't improve symptoms in 2–3 days
- You can't wear shoes comfortably
- This problem keeps coming back

Seek care right away if you have:

- **Diabetes**
- **Poor circulation**
- **Numbness in the feet**
- **Nerve damage** (neuropathy)

Even small infections can worsen quickly in these groups.

Your provider may recommend:

- Professional nail trimming or cleaning
- Partial removal of the ingrown portion
- Treatment for any infection
- A procedure to stop the nail edge from growing back inward
- Guidance on trimming and shoe selection

These procedures are usually done **in the office** and have a **high success rate** with proper follow-up.

Key Terms

- **Infection**: Swelling, redness, warmth, or drainage that can occur when skin is broken or irritated
- **Ingrown nail**: When the edge of a toenail grows into the surrounding skin
- **Nail matrix**: The area under the skin that produces the nail
- **Partial nail removal**: A procedure that removes only the problematic part of the nail
- **Toe box**: The front part of a shoe where the toes sit; narrow toe boxes increase risk

Notes:

Footnote Summary

- Ingrown toenails happen when the nail edge grows into the skin
- Soaking, wide shoes, and gentle care help mild cases
- Seek care if there is swelling, drainage, severe pain, or repeated ingrown nails

Athlete's Foot (Tinea Pedis)

What is it?

Athlete's foot is a **common fungal infection** that affects the skin on the feet—especially between the toes. It can cause itching, peeling, burning, and cracking of the skin.

You may notice:

- Itchy, red, or scaly skin
- Burning between the toes
- Blisters or peeling skin
- Dry, cracked skin on the bottom of the foot
- Strong or unpleasant foot odor

Athlete's foot is **not dangerous**, but it can spread to other toes, fingernails, or even the other foot if left untreated.

Why it happens

Athlete's foot is caused by **fungus** that grows in warm, damp places. It's common in people who sweat often, wear tight shoes, or walk barefoot in shared spaces.

Notes:

Common causes and risk factors include:

- Sweaty feet
- Wearing tight or closed shoes
- Walking barefoot in public showers, gyms, or pools
- Sharing shoes, socks, or towels
- Not fully drying the feet
- Reusing damp socks
- Toenail fungus (can spread to the skin)

What you can do at home

1. Keep your feet dry. Dry well between the toes after bathing. Moisture helps fungus grow.

2. Use antifungal creams or sprays. Apply daily for 2–4 weeks, even if symptoms begin to improve. Effective over-the-counter options include:

- Clotrimazole
- Terbinafine
- Miconazole

3. Change socks often. Avoid wearing the same shoes two days in a row. Wear moisture-wicking socks and change them:

- After exercise
- If they get damp
- At least once daily

4. Wear breathable shoes. Pick shoes that allow airflow, such as those with:

- Mesh material
- Ventilation holes
- A roomy toe box

5. Keep toenails trimmed. Fungus can hide under nails and spread to the skin.

6. Avoid sharing personal items. Do not share:

- Shoes
- Socks
- Towels
- Nail clippers

7. Treat your shoes. Spray or sprinkle **antifungal powder** inside shoes to kill leftover fungus and prevent reinfection.

When to seek care

See a specialist if:

- Symptoms last more than 2 weeks with treatment
- The skin cracks and becomes painful
- Redness or swelling spreads
- There is pus or signs of infection
- You have diabetes or poor circulation
- The infection keeps coming back

Cracked skin can lead to **secondary bacterial infections** in some cases.

Your provider may recommend:

- Stronger **prescription antifungal creams**
- Oral antifungal medication (for stubborn cases)
- Treatment of **toenail fungus**, if also present
- Evaluation for conditions that mimic athlete's foot (like **eczema** or **psoriasis**)

Notes:

Key Terms

- **Antifungal**: A medication that kills or slows the growth of fungus
- **Blistering**: Small fluid-filled bumps that can appear with skin irritation or infection
- **Moisture-wicking**: Fabric that pulls moisture away from the skin to help keep feet dry
- **Scaling**: Flaky or peeling skin, commonly seen in fungal infections
- **Tinea pedis**: The medical name for athlete's foot

Footnote Summary

- Athlete's foot is a fungal infection that causes itching, peeling, and burning skin.
- Keep feet dry, use antifungal creams, and rotate shoes.
- Seek care if symptoms last more than 2 weeks, infection spreads, or you have diabetes.

Toenail Fungus (Onychomycosis)

What is it?

Toenail fungus is an **infection of the nail**, often caused by the same type of fungus responsible for athlete's foot.

It usually starts at the tip of the nail and gradually spreads toward the base.

You may notice:

- Yellow, white, or brown spots on the nail
- Thick or brittle nails
- Nails that crumble or lift off the skin
- A foul smell
- Jagged or rough nail edges

The infection is **not dangerous**, but it can be **stubborn** and slow to treat.

Why it happens

According to **Mayo Clinic** and **Cleveland Clinic**, toenail fungus grows in **warm, moist** environments—like inside shoes.

Fungus enters through small cracks in the nail or nearby skin.

Common causes and risk factors include:

- Walking barefoot in public showers or pools
- Sweaty feet
- Tight or closed-toe shoes
- Athlete's foot that spreads to the nails
- Nail trauma
- Poor nail hygiene
- Aging (slower nail growth)
- Diabetes or poor circulation
- Weakened immune system

What you can do at home

1. Keep feet clean and dry. Wash and fully dry your feet every day, especially between the toes.

2. Trim nails straight across. Short, neatly trimmed nails reduce pressure and prevent nail trauma.

3. Use antifungal treatments. For mild cases, try consistent use of over-the-counter antifungal products such as:

- Antifungal creams
- Medicated nail lacquers
- Antifungal sprays

These may work for **mild** cases but require consistent use.

4. Rotate and air out shoes. Let shoes dry completely between wears. Avoid wearing the same pair two days in a row.

5. Wear breathable footwear. Look for shoes made of mesh or natural materials that allow airflow.

6. Change socks daily. Choose moisture-wicking socks and change them:

- After activity
- If damp
- At least once per day

7. Disinfect nail tools. Clean nail clippers and files after each use to avoid spreading fungus or reinfection.

When to seek care

See a specialist if:

- The nail becomes thick, painful, or deformed
- The nail lifts or separates from the skin
- More than one nail is affected
- Over-the-counter treatments are not working
- You have diabetes or poor circulation
- The fungus keeps coming back

Your provider may recommend:

- **Prescription antifungal pills** (most effective for stubborn infections)
- **Prescription nail lacquers**
- **Debridement** (in-office thinning of the nail)
- **Laser therapy** (available at some clinics)
- **Lab testing** to confirm fungal type

Note: Toenails grow slowly, so treatment may take **6 to 12 months** for full results.

Key Terms

- **Debridement** – Trimming or thinning a thickened toenail to reduce pressure and improve comfort
- **Fungus** – A living organism that thrives in warm, moist places and can infect skin or nails
- **Lacquer** – A medicated nail polish that delivers antifungal medication over time
- **Moisture-wicking socks** – Socks made to pull sweat away from the skin and keep feet dry
- **Onychomycosis** – The medical term for toenail fungus

Footnote Summary

- Toenail fungus causes thick, discolored, or crumbly nails
- Keep feet dry, use antifungal treatments, and rotate shoes
- Seek care if the nail is painful, very thick, or not improving

In summary

- *Skin and nail problems may seem small, but they can lead to discomfort and complications—especially if ignored.*
- *Conditions like **ingrown nails**, **fungal infections**, and **dry, cracked skin** often improve with proper hygiene, footwear, and early treatment.*
- *People with diabetes should check their feet regularly, as even minor issues can become serious.*

Notes:

H. Systemic & Circulation-Related

Finally, some foot and ankle problems are related to whole-body conditions, like diabetes or poor circulation. These issues can affect healing, nerve function, and overall foot health.

Diabetic Foot Problems (Especially Neuropathy)

What is it?

People with diabetes are more likely to develop **foot problems** because high blood sugar can damage:

- **Nerves**
- **Skin**
- **Circulation**
- **Healing ability**

The most serious complication is **diabetic neuropathy**, where the nerves in the feet do not work normally.

You may experience:

- Numbness or tingling
- Burning or shooting pain
- Loss of feeling
- Trouble sensing hot, cold, or pain

Because of this, small injuries can go unnoticed, increasing the risk of **infection, ulcers**, or **slow-healing wounds**.

Notes:

Other common diabetic foot issues include:

- Skin cracks
- Fungal infections
- Calluses
- Poor circulation
- Ulcers (open sores)
- Charcot foot (rare but serious bone damage)

Early care prevents most serious complications.

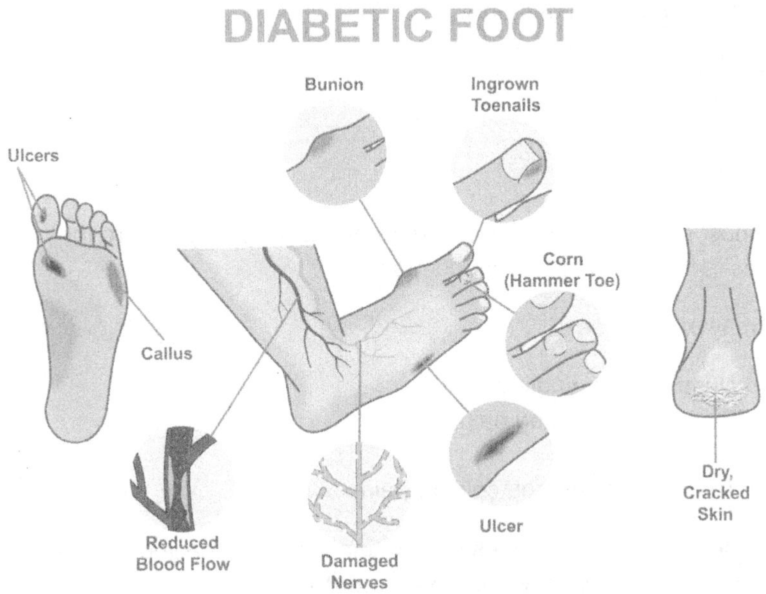

Why it happens

According to **Mayo Clinic** and the **American Diabetes Association**, diabetic foot problems result from long-term **high blood sugar** damaging nerves and blood vessels.

1. Nerve Damage (Neuropathy). High blood sugar injures the nerves in your feet. This leads to:

- Decreased sensation
- Poor pain awareness
- Muscle weakness or imbalance
- Balance problems

2. Poor Circulation. Diabetes narrows blood vessels, reducing blood flow to the feet. This slows healing and increases infection risk.

3. Skin Changes. Dry, cracked skin—especially around the heels—can create entry points for bacteria.

4. Weakened immune response. Diabetes can reduce the body's ability to fight infections and recover from injury.

What you can do at home

1. Check your feet every day. Use a mirror if needed. Look for:

- Redness
- Blisters
- Cuts
- Swelling
- Cracks
- Drainage
- Areas that feel "hot" or painful

2. Keep feet clean and dry

- Wash feet daily with warm (not hot) water
- Dry completely, especially between the toes

3. Moisturize (but not between the toes)

- Use lotion on tops and bottoms of feet
- Avoid moisture between toes (can lead to fungus)

4. Always wear protective shoes — even at home
Choose shoes that:

- Have a wide toe box
- Provide cushioning
- Do not rub or cause pressure

Avoid:

- Barefoot walking
- Flip-flops
- Thin slippers

5. Check shoes before putting them on. Neuropathy reduces your ability to feel objects. Check for:

- Rocks
- Folds in socks
- Foreign objects inside the shoe

6. Manage blood sugar. Maintaining your blood sugar is the **most important step** in protecting foot health.

7. Trim toenails safely.

- Trim straight across.
- Don't cut into corners.
- If you cannot see or reach well, ask a podiatrist

8. Treat fungus early. Athlete's foot and toenail fungus are common and can lead to infection.

9. Wear diabetic socks.

- Reduce pressure
- Wick moisture away
- Avoid tight bands around the calf

10. Try MEAT for mild pain

- **Movement** – Gentle range of motion
- **Exercise** – Light foot and ankle strength work
- **Analgesics** – If safe for you
- **Treatment** – Warm compresses (if not infected)

When to seek care

Seek *immediate* medical care if you notice:

- Open sores or ulcers
- Spreading redness
- Drainage or foul smell
- Sudden warmth in one area
- Black or blue skin changes
- Fever with foot wound
- Sharp increase in pain or numbness

See a specialist soon if:

- Tingling, burning, or numbness is new or worsening
- Skin cracks or sores do not heal
- New calluses develop
- Toenail fungus is spreading
- You can't feel the bottom of your foot well
- Shoes are causing pressure points

Good foot care can reduce the risk of foot ulcers and amputation by **up to 85%**.

Notes:

Your provider may recommend:

- Routine foot exams (every 3–12 months)
- Nerve testing (if neuropathy is suspected)
- Custom diabetic shoes or inserts
- Physical therapy for balance and strength
- Wound care (if ulcers are present)
- Imaging (X-ray or MRI for deeper infection)
- Blood flow studies

Key Terms

- **Callus**: Thickened skin from friction or pressure; can hide ulcers underneath in people with diabetes
- **Charcot foot**: A rare but serious condition where foot bones weaken, collapse, and deform
- **Diabetic shoes**: Specialized footwear to reduce pressure and prevent injury
- **Neuropathy**: Nerve damage that causes numbness, tingling, or burning
- **Ulcer**: A slow-healing open sore that requires close monitoring in diabetes

Footnote Summary

- **Neuropathy causes numbness or burning**, increasing injury risk
- **Check feet daily**, keep them clean and moisturized (but dry between toes)
- **Always wear protective shoes**
- **Seek care immediately** for ulcers, redness, swelling, or drainage

Peripheral Artery Disease (PAD)

What is it?

Peripheral Artery Disease (PAD) happens when arteries in the legs become **narrowed or clogged**, reducing blood flow to the **feet and ankles**. It's especially common in adults over 50—particularly those who **smoke**, have **diabetes**, or **high blood pressure**.

You may notice:

- Cramping or pain when walking (relieved by rest)
- Cold feet or legs
- Slow-healing cuts or sores
- Changes in skin color
- Brittle nails or hair loss on feet

Why it happens

According to **Mayo Clinic** and **Cleveland Clinic**, PAD is caused by **plaque buildup** (fat, cholesterol, and calcium) inside the arteries, which reduces oxygen delivery to the tissues—especially during activity.

Major causes and risk factors:

- **Smoking (the #1 cause)**
- **Diabetes**
- **High blood pressure**
- **High cholesterol**
- **Aging**
- **Kidney disease**
- **Family history**
- **Sedentary lifestyle**

Notes:

What you can do at home

1. Walk daily (even short distances)

- Use a “walk–rest–walk” pattern: walk until discomfort, rest, then walk again
- This improves circulation over time
- This improves circulation over time

2. Stop smoking

- Quitting is the **single most important step** to slow PAD progression

3. Manage health conditions

- Control **diabetes, blood pressure**, and **cholesterol** with medical guidance

4. Keep feet warm

- Wear socks and avoid walking barefoot—cold worsens symptoms

5. Moisturize dry skin

- Prevents cracks and lowers infection risk

6. Wear supportive shoes

- Avoid tight shoes that restrict circulation

7. Don’t cross your legs

- This can further reduce blood flow

Notes:

When to seek care

See a specialist if you notice:

- Pain in the feet or legs **while walking**
- Sores or cuts that heal slowly
- Cold feet or one foot colder than the other
- Color changes, brittle nails, or hair loss on the toes
- Numbness or tingling

Seek emergency care if:

- Your foot becomes blue, pale, or cold
- You suddenly can't move or feel your foot
- There's constant pain or blackened skin
  These may be signs of **critical limb ischemia**, a medical emergency.

Your provider may recommend:

- Pulse checks in the feet
- **ABI test** (ankle–brachial index)
- Vascular ultrasound or imaging
- Medications to improve blood flow
- Supervised walking program
- Referral to a **vascular specialist**
- In some cases, **procedures** to open or bypass blocked arteries

Notes:

Neuropathy vs. Radiculopathy: What's the Difference?

Symptom Pattern	Neuropathy (Foot Nerve)	Radiculopathy (Spine Nerve)
Pain location	Feet/toes	Starts in back or hip, travels down leg
Tingling/burning	Often in toes	Often down the leg
Worsens with	Standing/walking	Sitting or bending forward
Weakness	Usually foot only	May involve entire leg
Common cause	Diabetes, pressure	Herniated disc, stenosis
Best approach	Foot-focused treatment	Spine-focused treatment

Key Terms

- **ABI test** – A quick test comparing ankle and arm blood pressure to check circulation
- **Ischemia** – Lack of oxygen to tissue due to poor blood flow
- **PAD** – A condition where narrowed arteries reduce blood flow to legs and feet
- **Plaque** – Fat and cholesterol buildup inside arteries
- **Vascular** – Refers to blood vessels (arteries and veins)

Footnote Summary

- PAD reduces blood flow, causing pain and slow healing
- Walking programs, quitting smoking, and managing diabetes help improve symptoms
- Seek care for **slow-healing wounds**, **cold feet**, or **pain with walking**

In summary

- *Some foot and ankle problems are signs of whole-body conditions like diabetes or circulation disorders.*
- *These can affect healing, nerves, and tissue health—and require special care.*
- *Daily foot checks, good blood sugar control, proper footwear, and prompt attention to sores or numbness can prevent serious complications.*

Notes:

PAIN PATTERN CHART: What Your Pain Location Might Mean

Pain Location	Possible Cause(s)	Typical Clues You May Notice
Bottom of the heel	Plantar fasciitis	Worst with first steps in the morning; sharp, stabbing pain
Arch of the foot	Plantar fasciitis, flat feet, overuse strain	Achy pain after standing/walking; improves with supportive shoes
Outside of the foot / ankle	Peroneal tendonitis, ankle sprain, 5th metatarsal stress fracture	Pain with uneven ground; swelling after activity
Inside of the ankle	Posterior tibial tendonitis, flatfoot changes, tarsal tunnel	Pain with standing; arch seems to collapse; possible tingling
Back of the heel	Achilles tendonitis	Pain when walking uphill or climbing stairs; stiffness in the morning
Front of the ankle	Impingement, arthritis	Pain when bending ankle upward or squatting
Ball of the foot	Metatarsalgia, neuroma, hammertoe pressure	Burning or tingling; worsens in tight shoes
Big toe joint	Arthritis, bunion, gout	Pain with push-off; swelling/redness possible
Middle of foot (top)	Stress fracture, midfoot sprain	Sharp pain with walking; swelling; pain touching the top of foot
Toes (burning or numbness)	Neuropathy, Morton's neuroma	Tingling, burning, or "sock bunched up" feeling

Top 10 Mistakes Patients Make With Foot & Ankle Pain

1. Ignoring pain for weeks instead of addressing it early
2. Wearing worn-out shoes with poor support
3. Walking or running through pain, worsening the injury
4. Not stretching calves, which contribute to most heel and arch problems
5. Relying only on rest, without strengthening or mobility work
6. Skipping supportive footwear at home (barefoot on hard floors)
7. Overusing braces or boots when not medically necessary
8. Using Dr. Google and misdiagnosing themselves
9. Stopping treatment too soon once pain improves

Not following up after injuries, especially ankle sprains that feel "better enough" but heal incorrectly

Notes:

Notes:

SECTION 4

Diagnosis & Testing

What to expect during your exam and how providers make a diagnosis.

What Happens During the Exam

- During your visit, your medical provider will do a hands-on exam of your foot and ankle
- This helps them figure out which bones, tendons, nerves, or joints are causing your symptoms
- The exam is gentle, and you can tell the provider at any time if something hurts

1. Looking at your foot (Inspection)

Your provider will begin by looking at both feet, comparing the painful side to the healthy one. This helps identify visible patterns that match certain conditions. They will check for:

- Swelling
- Redness or bruising
- Changes in skin color
- Changes in nail appearance
- Calluses or pressure spots
- Arch shape (flat feet or high arches)
- Toe alignment (bunions, hammertoes, drifting toes)
- Heel position (tilted in or out)
- How you stand

2. Feeling the foot (Palpation)

Next, the provider will gently press on different areas to find the exact spot of pain. This helps narrow down which structure is irritated, such as a tendon, ligament, or joint. They may press on:

- The heel and arch
- The ball of the foot
- Each toe joint
- The Achilles tendon
- The inside and outside of the ankle
- Ligaments and soft tissue areas

3. Range of motion (How Your Foot Moves)

Your provider will move your foot and ankle in different directions:

- Up (dorsiflexion)
- Down (plantarflexion)
- Inward (inversion)
- Outward (eversion)
- Toe bending

They check:

- How far the joint moves
- Whether movement causes pain
- If the joint feels tight or stiff

This tells them whether the problem is in the joint, tendon, or muscle.

4. Strength testing. Weakness helps identify nerve problems or tendon injuries. You may be asked to push or pull against the provider's hand. This checks:

- Muscle strength
- Tendon function
- Whether certain movements increase pain

Examples:

- Pushing the foot down (tests calf and Achilles)
- Pulling the foot up (tests anterior tibialis)
- Turning the foot inward or outward (tests ankle tendons)
- Lifting the big toe (tests specific nerves)

5. Walking and balance tests. This helps show how the injury affects daily movement. Your provider may watch you:

- Walk normally
- Walk on heels
- Walk on toes
- Stand on one foot
- Do a small squat or step

They look for:

- Limping
- Guarding
- Differences between sides
- Problems with balance
- Signs of nerve weakness

6. Ligament stability tests. These gentle tests help check for sprains. They also help diagnose ankle sprains and chronic ankle instability. Your provider may:

- Move the foot side to side
- Tug gently on the ankle joint
- Check how much the ligament stretches

These tests can show if a ligament is:

- Irritated
- Stretched
- Partially torn
- Fully torn

7. Tendon tests. Each tendon has a specific job. Your provider may:

- Press along the tendon
- Ask you to move the foot while they resist
- Check for swelling, warmth, or pain

This helps diagnose problems like:

- Achilles tendonitis
- Peroneal tendonitis
- Posterior tibial tendon dysfunction
- Extensor tendonitis

Notes:

8. Nerve checks. Your provider may test nerves by checking:

- Light touch sensation
- Reflexes
- Toe lifting strength
- Tapping along nerve pathways

These tests help detect:

- Tarsal tunnel syndrome
- Lumbar radiculopathy
- Morton's neuroma
- Diabetic neuropathy

9. Circulation check. Your provider may check the pulses in your foot and compare both sides. This helps screen for circulation problems or Peripheral Artery Disease (PAD). They may also look at:

- Skin temperature
- Hair growth
- Nail changes
- Color changes

10. Special tests (Only If Needed). These help confirm or rule out specific diagnoses. Depending on your symptoms, the provider may perform simple, targeted tests:

- **Drawer test** – A test where the provider moves the foot forward and back to check the stability of the ankle ligaments
- **Mulder click test** – A test that squeezes the forefoot to check for Morton's neuroma; a "click" may be felt
- **Single-leg heel raise** – An exercise/test where you lift your heel while standing on one leg to check the strength of the posterior tibial tendon
- **Squeeze test** – A test where the provider squeezes the leg bones together to check for a possible stress fracture
- **Thompson test** – A test where the provider squeezes the calf muscle to see if the Achilles tendon is intact
- **Tinel's sign** – A test where the provider taps over a nerve to check for irritation or tingling

🩺 ***Surgeons note:*** *" I am looking at many things during this exam: I look at both feet, standing and walking. I check how your foot moves, where it hurts, and how your body compensates. I will ask you to walk normally, walk on your tip toes, walk on your heels, and I will test your sensation also."*

Footnote Summary

- The exam includes looking, touching, moving, and testing the foot and ankle
- Your provider checks strength, motion, nerves, joints, and circulation
- These simple tests help identify which structure is injured or irritated
- You can speak up at any time if something hurts

Notes:

Weight-Bearing vs. Non-Weight-Bearing Imaging

Why Imaging Matters

When your provider orders X-rays, MRIs, or other scans, they may choose **weight-bearing** or **non-weight-bearing** imaging—or both. Each type gives **different information** about how your foot and ankle look and function. This section explains what they are, when they're used, and why both may be needed for a full diagnosis.

What Are Weight-Bearing Images?

Weight-bearing imaging is done while you're **standing** and your **foot is supporting your body weight**—just like during walking or daily activity.

This helps show:

- How bones align under pressure
- The true shape of your **arch**
- **Joint movement** and function while standing
- Instability or collapse not seen at rest
- Changes that only happen during weight-bearing

Especially helpful for:

- Flat feet or fallen arches
- High arches
- Bunions and hammertoes
- Midfoot arthritis
- Toe alignment issues
- Ankle arthritis
- Post-injury instability

Some conditions only appear **when the foot is loaded**, so this test shows a more accurate picture of your real-life foot mechanics.

What Are Non-Weight-Bearing Images?

Non-weight-bearing imaging is done while you're **sitting or lying down**, with no pressure on the foot.

Often used for:

- **X-rays** when weight-bearing is too painful
- **MRI**, **CT**, or **ultrasound**
- Getting a detailed view of internal structures at rest

These scans show:

- Bone structure and alignment
- Joint spacing
- Fractures
- Ligament or tendon tears
- Swelling or fluid buildup
- Soft tissue problems (depending on the test)

Why Your Provider May Order Both

Weight-bearing and non-weight-bearing tests show **different aspects** of the same problem.

- **Weight-bearing** = function, alignment under pressure
- **Non-weight-bearing** = structure, soft tissues, inflammation

Together, they provide:

- A full view of **joint health** and **alignment**
- Insight into **soft tissue injuries**
- Information on how **standing affects your foot**
- A more confident diagnosis

Notes:

Non-Weight-Bearing Imaging Is Most Helpful For:

- Stress fractures
- Sesamoiditis
- Ligament injuries
- Tendonitis or tendon tears
- Heel pain
- Swelling or fluid collection
- Bone bruises or inflammation

What to Expect During the Test

Weight-Bearing X-rays

- You'll stand on a platform
- The technician will position your foot
- You'll hold still briefly
- The process is quick and painless

Non-Weight-Bearing Imaging

- You'll sit or lie down
- The foot is gently positioned
- The process is comfortable and noninvasive
- MRI or CT may take longer but are also painless

Footnote Summary

- **Weight-bearing imaging** shows how your foot functions under real-life pressure
- **Non-weight-bearing imaging** shows bones and soft tissues at rest
- Your provider may order **both** to get the most accurate diagnosis and treatment plan

Notes:

SECTION 5

Non-Surgical Treatments

Practical treatments that help most people improve without surgery.

RICE vs. MEAT

When you first hurt your foot or ankle, it can be confusing to know whether to **rest** or **start moving**. Two common guides—**RICE** and **MEAT**—can help.

Both are useful, but they are meant for **different stages** of healing.

What Is RICE?

RICE is used right after an injury to reduce swelling and protect the area.

- **R** – Rest
- **I** – Ice
- **C** – Compression
- **E** – Elevation

Use RICE if you have:

- A **new injury**
- **Swelling** or **bruising**
- **Sharp pain** with walking
- A **sprain, strain, or trauma**
- Pain that worsens with activity

How RICE Helps:

- **Rest**: Prevents further damage
- **Ice**: Reduces swelling and pain
- **Compression**: Controls fluid buildup
- **Elevation**: Helps drain fluid away from the foot

⏱ Most people use RICE for the **first 24–72 hours** after an acute injury.

Notes:

What Is MEAT?

MEAT helps after the swelling has gone down and the injury is starting to heal.

- **M** – Movement
- **E** – Exercise
- **A** – Analgesics (pain relief, if safe)
- **T** – Treatment (like heat, massage, or hands-on care)

Use **MEAT** when:

- Swelling is **improving**
- Pain feels more like **stiffness** than sharp pain
- You can **walk with less limping**
- You are **past the first few days**
- Your provider says it's **safe to move**

How MEAT Helps:

- **Movement**: Prevents stiffness
- **Exercise**: Slowly restores strength
- **Analgesics**: Help reduce pain so you can move
- **Treatment**: Heat or massage improves circulation

When to Use Each

Choose RICE if:

- You just injured your foot or ankle
- It is **painful to bear weight**
- You have **visible swelling or bruising**
- Pain gets **worse with motion**

Choose **MEAT** if:

- Swelling has gone down
- Pain feels **dull or stiff**, not sharp
- You're **starting to walk better**
- You're in the **healing phase**

Most patients move from **RICE** → **MEAT** over several days as healing begins.

Common Mistakes to Avoid

❌ Too much rest → can cause stiffness or weakness

❌ Too much early movement → may worsen swelling

❌ Walking through sharp pain → may delay healing

❌ Skipping rehab exercises → slows recovery

❌ Using heat too early → can increase swelling

Bonus Tip: Protecting Your Feet on Vacation

- ☐ Wear **supportive shoes** at airports
- ☐ **Bring your brace** if you use one
- ☐ Don't break in **new shoes** on a trip
- ☐ Avoid **barefoot walking on sand** if you have **tendonitis**
- ☐ ❌ Never walk barefoot on sand if you have **neuropathy** – you may not feel burns or cuts
- ☐ **Elevate** your feet when you return to the hotel
- ☐ Pack a **travel ice pack**

Key Terms

- **Acute injury**: A new or sudden injury
- **Analgesic**: A medicine that relieves pain
- **Circulation**: Blood flow that helps healing
- **Stiffness**: Tightness or reduced motion in a joint
- **Swelling**: Fluid buildup that causes puffiness

Footnote Summary

- Use **RICE** in the **first 24–72 hours** after an injury to reduce pain and swelling
- Switch to **MEAT** as symptoms improve to rebuild motion and strength
- RICE protects the area; MEAT helps it recover
- Your provider can help you know when to switch from RICE to MEAT

What NOT to Do

Avoid these common mistakes during foot or ankle recovery:

❌ Don't push through **severe pain**

❌ Don't ignore **swelling** that doesn't improve

❌ Don't sleep in a **brace** unless told to

❌ Don't "Google diagnose" your injury

❌ Don't do **aggressive stretching** after a new injury

❌ Don't go **barefoot** if you have **neuropathy**

❌ Don't delay **imaging** if pain lasts more than 2 weeks after injury

Notes:

Braces, Boots & Splints

Understanding the devices your provider may recommend

Foot and ankle injuries often need extra support while healing. **Braces, boots, splints, and offloading devices** help reduce pain, support weak tissues, and prevent further damage.

Why Support Devices Are Helpful

Support devices are used when the foot or ankle is:

- Weak
- Swollen
- Unstable
- Painful to walk on
- At risk for further damage

They help by:

- Reducing movement
- Supporting ligaments and tendons
- Maintaining proper joint position
- Reducing pain during daily activity
- Allowing healing without surgery

Your provider will select the right device based on your specific injury.

1. Ankle Braces

Used for sprains, strains, tendon irritation, and instability.

Common Types:

- **Elastic sleeves**: Light support for swelling or mild sprains
- **Lace-up braces**: Limit side-to-side movement, good for instability
- **Figure-8 braces**: Extra ligament support
- **Rigid ankle braces**: Plastic sides prevent ankle rolling

Why They're Used:

- Support healing ligaments
- Reduce swelling
- Prevent ankle rolling
- Help with chronic instability

Patient Tips:

- Wear with socks to prevent skin irritation
- Ensure the brace is snug but not too tight
- Can be used during walking or sports

2. Walking Boots (CAM Boots)

Used for fractures, tendon injuries, and severe sprains.

Common Types:

- **Tall boot**: For ankle or Achilles injuries
- **Short boot**: For foot fractures or forefoot pain
- **Rocker-bottom boot**: Helps with smoother walking while protected

Why They're Used:

- Stabilize fractures
- Reduce pain
- Allow partial/full weight-bearing
- Protect healing ligaments and tendons
- Reduce pressure on the forefoot

Patient Tips:

- Use a **heel lift** in the opposite shoe to prevent hip/back pain
- Wear **long socks** to protect your skin
- Keep the boot on unless told otherwise
- **Do not drive** in a boot unless cleared by your provider

3. Splints

Used for acute injuries, nighttime support, or toe problems.

Common Types:

- **Night splints**: Stretch calf and plantar fascia during sleep

- **Posterior splints**: Stabilize back of foot/ankle
- **Toe splints**: Help straighten injured or crooked toes
- **Post-op splints**: Used after surgery

Why They're Used:

- Reduce movement during early healing
- Keep tendons stretched (e.g., plantar fascia)
- Protect joints during rest or sleep
- Support soft tissues after injury

Patient Tips:

- Night splints should feel snug—not painful
- Take breaks if skin becomes irritated
- Don't modify splints yourself—ask your provider

4. Offloading Devices

Used for plantar fasciitis, forefoot injuries, sesamoiditis, and ulcers.

Examples:

- Offloading shoes
- Forefoot relief shoes
- Dancer's pads (for sesamoids)
- Heel cups
- Pressure-relieving wedges

Why They're Used:

- Shift pressure away from painful areas
- Help protect stress fractures
- Reduce pain from sesamoid or plantar plate injuries

Patient Tips:

- Follow placement instructions from your provider
- Some pads go **behind** the painful spot, not on it

5. When Are These NOT Appropriate?

Avoid using braces, boots, or splints if:

- They cause **increased pain**
- You have **circulation issues** (e.g., PAD)
- You have **neuropathy** and cannot feel your foot
- There is **skin breakdown** or **infection**
- The device increases **fall risk**

Always follow your provider's recommendations.

6. How Long Will I Wear Them?

Usually **2–6 weeks**, depending on:

- The severity of the injury
- Type of device used
- Your progress during healing
- Your provider will adjust the plan as you recover.

🩺 **Surgeon's Note:** "Use braces exactly as directed — no more, no less.

- Wear socks to protect your skin, and inspect daily for redness or pressure spots.
- **Too much bracing** leads to weakness.
- **Too little bracing** delays healing.
- Follow your provider's instructions closely."

When Orthotics Help — and When They Don't

Based on AAOS.org, American Orthopaedic Foot & Ankle Society (AOFAS), and national orthotics guidance

Orthotics (shoe inserts or arch supports) can be a helpful part of foot and ankle treatment—but they are not a fix-all. This section explains when they're useful and when they're unlikely to help.

When Orthotics Help

Orthotics are often helpful if you have:

- Flat feet causing arch strain or **posterior tibial tendonitis**
- **Plantar fasciitis** that improves with arch support
- Mild-to-moderate **bunions** or **hammertoes** needing pressure relief
- Arthritis in the **midfoot** or **big toe** where cushioning reduces pain
- Long hours of **standing or walking** that require shock absorption
- **High arches** that lack natural shock absorption

In these cases, orthotics can provide support, reduce strain, and improve comfort during daily activities.

When Orthotics Do Not Help

National guidelines note that orthotics are **less effective** if:

- Pain is caused by a **stress fracture**
- You have an **acute injury** (sudden sprain, swelling)
- There is a **complete tendon tear** (which may require bracing or surgery)
- Pain is from **nerve compression** (like **neuropathy** or **tarsal tunnel syndrome**)
- Your footwear can't accommodate orthotics (e.g., flip-flops or high heels)
- You rely on orthotics alone, without doing stretching or strengthening

Summary:
Orthotics support the foot but don't heal structural injuries. They work best when combined with proper shoes, stretching, strengthening, and activity modification.

Key Terms

- **Offloading**: Shifting pressure away from a painful area to help it heal
- **Rocker-bottom sole**: A curved shoe sole that allows smoother walking and reduces forefoot pressure
- **Splint**: A rigid support used short-term to reduce painful motion
- **Stabilization**: Limiting joint movement to allow tissues to heal
- **Walking boot (CAM boot)**: A removable boot that limits motion and protects the foot or ankle during healing

Footnote Summary

- **Braces, boots, splints, and orthotics** support healing and reduce pain
- Use each device for the **right injury** at the **right time**
- **Orthotics** help with support problems—not fractures or severe tears
- Always follow your provider's guidance on **how long to wear** these devices and **what to wear them with**

Notes:

Physical Therapy, Occupational Therapy & Home Exercises

- **Rebuilding strength, flexibility, and confidence in your feet**
- Physical therapy (PT), occupational therapy (OT), and consistent home exercises play a major role in helping your foot or ankle heal.
- These treatments improve motion, restore strength, and help you return to normal activities more safely and confidently.

Why Therapy Helps:

Physical Therapy (PT) helps with:

- Improving strength
- Restoring motion
- Reducing pain
- Training balance
- Correcting walking patterns
- Protecting healing tissues

PT is especially helpful for:

- Ankle sprains
- Plantar fasciitis
- Achilles problems
- Tendonitis
- Arthritis
- After wearing a boot or cast
- After surgery

Notes:

Occupational Therapy (OT)

OT focuses on staying safe and independent, especially for older adults or those with mobility concerns. OT is helpful when foot or ankle pain affects:

- Walking around the house
- Climbing stairs
- Bathing, dressing, or other daily tasks
- Balance and stability
- Home safety

OT may recommend:

- Fall prevention strategies
- Assistive devices (cane, walker, sock aid, grab bars)
- Changes in the home environment (rugs, chairs, bathroom setup)

What to Expect During Therapy

During sessions, your therapist will assess:

- Strength
- Flexibility
- Range of motion
- Pain level
- Balance
- Walking pattern

Treatment may include:

- Stretching
- Strength training
- Soft tissue work or massage
- Joint mobilization
- Balance exercises
- Gait (walking) training
- Ice or heat
- Taping or bracing
- Dry needling (some clinics)

Therapy **should not be extremely painful.** Mild soreness is normal, but stop if something feels sharp or wrong.

Common Foot & Ankle Home Exercises

Always ask your provider before starting new exercises—especially after a fracture, surgery, or if you're wearing a brace or boot.

Stretching Exercises

1. Calf Stretch (Wall Stretch)

- Face a wall and step one foot back
- Keep the back knee straight
- Lean forward
- Hold for 20–30 seconds
- Repeat 3–5 times

Helps: plantar fasciitis, Achilles issues, flat feet

2. Plantar Fascia Stretch (Towel Stretch)

- Sit with your leg straight
- Loop a towel around the ball of your foot
- Pull gently toward you
- Hold for 20–30 seconds
- Repeat 3–5 times

Helps: heel pain, arch pain

3. Toe Extension Stretch

- Sit and cross your leg
- Gently pull your big toe upward
- Hold for 20 seconds
- Repeat 3–5 times

Helps: hallux rigidus, plantar fasciitis

Strengthening Exercises

1. Towel Curls

- Sit and place a towel under your foot
- Curl your toes to pull the towel toward you
- Repeat 10–15 times

Helps: toe strength, arch control

2. Marble Pick-Up

- Place marbles on the floor
- Pick them up using your toes
- Drop them into a small cup or bowl

Helps: toe control, neuromuscular coordination

3. Ankle Alphabet

- Sit with your foot elevated
- "Draw" the alphabet in the air with your foot
- Use slow, smooth motion

Helps: ankle motion, recovery after sprains

4. Heel Raises

- Stand near a counter
- Rise up on your toes, then slowly lower
- Start with both legs, then progress to one

Helps: calf strength, Achilles rehab

Notes:

5. Resistance Band Ankle Work

- Use a resistance band to strengthen:
    - Upward motion (dorsiflexion)
    - Downward motion (plantarflexion)
    - Inward turning (inversion)
    - Outward turning (eversion)

Helps: sprains, instability, tendonitis

Balance & Stability Exercises

1. Single-Leg Stand

- Stand on one foot
- Hold for 20–30 seconds
- For a challenge: close your eyes or stand on a soft surface

Helps: balance, ankle control

2. Heel-to-Toe Walk

- Walk in a straight line
- Place one foot directly in front of the other (heel to toe)

Helps: stability, gait training

Functional Exercises

When strength and motion improve, your therapist may add:

- Step-ups
- Gentle squats or lunges
- Walking drills
- Stair training
- Sport-specific movements

These exercises help you safely return to daily life or athletic activities.

When to Stop or Modify Exercises

Stop and contact your provider or therapist if you have:

- Sharp pain
- Sudden swelling
- Numbness or tingling
- Pain that lasts more than 24–48 hours
- Feeling of "giving way" or instability

Mild muscle soreness is normal—but **pain that gets worse** is not.

Key Terms

- **Balance training**: Exercises that improve stability and reduce fall risk
- **Mobility**: Ability of a joint to move through its full range
- **OT (Occupational Therapy)**: Therapy focused on safe, independent movement in daily life
- **PT (Physical Therapy)**: Therapy focused on motion, strength, and injury recovery
- **Strengthening**: Building muscle to support joints and protect from injury

Footnote Summary

- **Movement is medicine**: Gentle exercise supports healing better than rest alone
- **Strength matters**: Strong muscles protect joints, tendons, and prevent re-injury
- **Balance improves safety**: Small balance exercises reduce fall risk and build confidence
- **Therapists are guides**: PTs and OTs teach you how to move, stretch, and recover safely
- **Daily practice helps you heal**: A few minutes of stretching and strengthening can make a big difference

Medications for Ankle & Foot Pain

Medication can help reduce **pain and swelling** while your foot or ankle heals.

Most medications **do not fix the root cause**, but they can make it easier to move, stretch, and recover—especially in the early or painful phases of an injury.

This section explains the **main types of medications** your provider may recommend, when to use them, and what to watch out for.

1. NSAIDs (Non-Steroidal Anti-Inflammatory Drugs).

NSAIDs help by reducing both:

- **Pain**
- **Swelling (inflammation)**

They are often used short-term for **acute injuries**, sprains, or flare-ups of chronic conditions like arthritis or tendonitis.

NSAIDs work best for:

- Sprains and strains
- Tendonitis
- Plantar fasciitis
- Arthritis
- Pain with swelling
- Acute injuries (not fractures)

⚠ **Important:** NSAIDs may **not be safe** for everyone. Use caution or avoid if you:

- Have **kidney problems**
- Have **stomach ulcers**
- Take **blood thinners**
- Have **heart issues**

Always check with your provider or pharmacist before starting an NSAID regularly.

Common NSAIDs for Foot and Ankle Pain

Generic Name	Brand Name	What It Helps	Common Side Effects
Ibuprofen	Advil, Motrin	Pain, swelling, inflammation	Stomach upset, heartburn
Naproxen	Aleve	Long-lasting relief for sprains & tendonitis	Stomach irritation, dizziness
Meloxicam	Mobic	Arthritis, chronic inflammation	Upset stomach, swelling, headache
Celecoxib	Celebrex	Arthritis, (gentler on stomach for some)	Indigestion, swelling, possible rash

Note: Prescription NSAIDs may be stronger or longer-acting. Your provider will help choose the right one for your needs.

2. Acetaminophen (Tylenol)

Acetaminophen helps relieve **pain**, but **does not reduce swelling** like NSAIDs do. Best for:

- Mild to moderate pain
- Pain after injury
- People who **cannot take NSAIDs** (due to stomach, kidney, or heart issues)

⚠ **Important Safety Notes:**

- Generally well-tolerated
- Rarely causes stomach upset
- **High doses can damage the liver**
  → Do not exceed 3,000mg per day (including combination medications)
  → Ask your provider if you have liver disease or take other medications that affect the liver

3. Nerve Pain Medicines

These medicines are designed to treat **nerve-related symptoms**, such as:

- Burning
- Tingling
- Numbness
- Radiating pain
- Electric-shock feelings

They **do not work immediately**—they usually take **1–3 weeks** to start helping.

Often used for:

- Diabetic neuropathy
- Tarsal tunnel syndrome
- Lumbar radiculopathy
- Nerve compression or irritation

Common Nerve Pain Medicines

Generic Name	Brand Name	What It Helps	Common Side Effects
Gabapentin	Neurontin	Nerve pain, tingling, burning	Sleepiness, dizziness
Pregabalin	Lyrica	Nerve pain, neuropathy	Drowsiness, swelling, weight gain
Duloxetine	Cymbalta	Nerve pain + mood support	Nausea, dry mouth, fatigue
Amitriptyline	Elavil	Nerve pain, nighttime pain	Drowsiness, dry mouth, constipation

4. **Opioids** (Short-Term Only) help with severe pain right after:

- A major injury
- Surgery
- A fracture

They are used short-term only, usually just a few days.

Important Safety Notes:

- They cause constipation — take a bowel regimen
- Never mix with alcohol or sedating medications
- Risk of dependence increases with long-term use
- Not recommended for chronic foot and ankle pain

Common Opioids

Generic Name	Brand Name	What It Helps	Common Side Effects
Hydrocodone + acetaminophen	Norco, Vicodin	Severe, short-term pain	Constipation, drowsiness
Oxycodone	Roxicodone	Post-surgical or fracture pain	Nausea, dizziness
Tramadol	Ultram	Moderate to severe pain	Headache, sleepiness, nausea

5. Topical Medications

Topical medications are **creams, gels, or patches** applied directly to the painful area. They work **locally**, which means **less risk of stomach, kidney, or heart side effects** than oral medications.

Topicals are especially helpful for people who:

- **Cannot take NSAIDs** by mouth
- Have **mild to moderate pain**
- Need relief in a **specific area**
- Want to **avoid systemic side effects**

Common Topicals

Generic / Type	Brand Name	What It Helps	Common Side Effects
Diclofenac gel	Voltaren	Arthritis, tendonitis, foot pain	Mild skin irritation
Lidocaine patch/cream	Lidoderm, Aspercreme	Nerve pain, burning, tender areas	Numbness, skin redness
Capsaicin cream	Capzasin, Zostrix	Nerve pain (after regular use)	Burning or warmth sensation
Menthol/methyl salicylate	Biofreeze, Icy Hot	Temporary relief of ache or soreness	Cooling or warming sensation

▲ Tips for Use

- Wash hands after applying
- Avoid applying over broken skin or open wounds
- Do not use heat (like heating pads) over the area after applying
- Effects may vary — capsaicin works best after regular use for 1–2 weeks

6. Adjuvant Medications (SNRIs, TCAs)

These medications are **originally used for mood or sleep**, but they are also **very effective for nerve and chronic pain**—especially when pain has lasted longer than 3 months.

They work by calming nerve signals in the brain and spinal cord.

These medications are often helpful for:

- Burning or shooting pain
- Pain that **interrupts sleep**
- **Diabetic neuropathy**
- Long-term pain that does not respond to other medications

⚠ These do **not work immediately** — they may take **2–4 weeks** to show results

-Often taken at night to reduce side effects like drowsiness

Common Adjuvant Medications

Generic Name	Brand Name	Medication Type	What It Helps	Common Side Effects
Duloxetine	Cymbalta	SNRI	Nerve pain, chronic pain, mood	Nausea, dry mouth
Venlafaxine	Effexor	SNRI	Nerve pain, chronic pain	Sweating, dizziness
Amitriptyline	Elavil	TCA	Nighttime nerve pain	Drowsiness, dry mouth
Nortriptyline	Pamelor	TCA	Neuropathy, sleep-related pain	Constipation, dizziness

7. What to Tell Your Provider Before Starting Any Medication

Before starting any new medication, make sure to tell your provider about:

- All medications you currently take (including prescription, over-the-counter, supplements, and herbs)
- Any history of **stomach ulcers**, GI bleeding, or acid reflux
- **Kidney or liver problems**
- **Alcohol use** (even occasional)
- **Sleep issues** or fatigue
- **Numbness, tingling**, or nerve-related symptoms
- **Medication allergies** or sensitivities
- If you are **pregnant, planning to become pregnant, or breastfeeding**

This helps your provider choose the safest and most effective treatment plan.

Key Terms

- **Acetaminophen**: A common over-the-counter pain reliever that helps reduce pain but not inflammation
- **Adjuvant medications**: Medicines originally used for mood or sleep that also help nerve and chronic pain
- **Analgesic**: A medication that helps relieve pain
- **Capsaicin**: A chili pepper extract used in creams to reduce nerve pain over time
- **Diclofenac**: A topical anti-inflammatory used to treat arthritis or tendon pain
- **Gabapentin**: A nerve pain medication that reduces burning, tingling, and electric-shock sensations
- **Lidocaine**: A numbing medication used in patches or creams to calm painful or irritated nerves
- **NSAIDs (Non-Steroidal Anti-Inflammatory Drugs)** – A group of medicines that reduce both pain and inflammation
- **Opioids**: Strong pain relievers meant for short-term use only because they can be habit-forming
- **SNRIs/TCAs**: Medications that can help with chronic or nerve pain by affecting how the brain processes pain signals
- **Topicals**: Creams, gels, or patches placed on the skin to relieve pain in a specific area

Footnote Summary

- Different medications help different types of foot and ankle pain
- **NSAIDs** help with inflammation; **acetaminophen** helps with general pain
- **Nerve pain medications** calm tingling, burning, or numbness
- **Opioids** are for short-term use only, usually after injury or surgery
- **Topicals** are a great option if oral medications cause side effects
- Always follow your provider's instructions and report any new or worsening symptoms

Injections & Procedures

Options to reduce pain and support healing

Some foot and ankle problems respond well to office-based injections or procedures. These treatments can reduce inflammation, relieve pain, and help your provider target the exact area of concern.

1. PRP (Platelet-Rich Plasma)

What it is: Uses your own blood platelets to stimulate healing

How it works:

- Blood is drawn and spun in a centrifuge
- Platelets are concentrated and injected into the injured area

Best for:

- Chronic tendonitis (Achilles, peroneal, posterior tibial)
- Plantar fasciitis
- Mild to moderate arthritis
- Slow-healing injuries

Pros: Natural, uses your own cells, fewer side effects

Cons: Not covered by insurance, may take 2–3 months and multiple injections to notice improvement

Common side effects: Mild soreness, temporary swelling

2. Steroid (Corticosteroid) Injections

What it is: Anti-inflammatory medicine injected into painful areas

How it works: Often mixed with numbing medication for fast relief; steroid works over several days

Best for:

- Arthritis (ankle, midfoot, big toe)
- Plantar fasciitis
- Tendonitis
- Morton's neuroma
- Bursitis or acute flare-ups

Pros: Fast relief, reduces swelling, helps confirm diagnosis

Cons: Can't be repeated too often

Side effects: Temporary soreness, swelling, facial flushing, blood sugar rise (diabetics)

3. Joint Injections

What it is: Delivers medication into a specific joint

Used for:

- Ankle, subtalar, or midfoot arthritis
- Big toe arthritis (hallux rigidus)

Medication used:

- Steroids (most common)
- PRP (in some clinics)
- Hyaluronic acid (less common)

Pros: Reduces inflammation and pain, may improve joint movement

Side effects: Soreness, rare infection, sugar spikes

Notes:

4. Tendon Sheath Injections

What it is: Injection around the tendon lining (not the tendon itself)

Used for:

- Trigger toe
- Peroneal, posterior tibial, or flexor tendonitis

Benefits: Calms irritation, improves tendon gliding

Risks: Soreness, flare-ups, tendon weakening if repeated

5. Nerve Blocks

What it is: Numbing medicine around a nerve

Used for:

- Morton's neuroma
- Tarsal tunnel (diagnostic or therapeutic)
- Nerve pain from injury or compression

How it helps:

- Temporary relief
- Can identify the exact nerve involved

Side effects: Temporary numbness, mild weakness, bruising

6. Ultrasound- or X-Ray-Guided Injections

Why it's used:

- Improves accuracy
- Reduces risk of hitting the wrong structure
- Helps reach small or deep targets in the foot and ankle

7. What to Expect After an Injection

You may experience:

- Numbness for a few hours
- Mild soreness for 1–2 days
- Temporary flare-up of pain
- Gradual relief over a few days to weeks

Avoid heavy activity the day of the injection unless told otherwise.

8. When Injections Are *Not* Recommended

Injections may be avoided if you have:

- Active skin or joint infection
- Open wounds near the site
- Poorly controlled diabetes (for steroids)
- Certain tendon tears (risk of further weakening)
- Bleeding disorders

Each decision is made on a case-by-case basis.

Key Terms

- **Corticosteroid**: A strong anti-inflammatory medication that reduces swelling and pain
- **Hyaluronic acid**: A gel-like substance sometimes injected into joints to improve lubrication
- **Injection**: Delivering medication directly into a joint, tendon, or tissue
- **Nerve block**: Injection that numbs a nerve to reduce or diagnose pain
- **Platelet-Rich Plasma (PRP)**: A treatment using concentrated platelets from your own blood to promote healing
- **Tendon sheath**: The protective lining that surrounds a tendon and helps it glide smoothly
- **Ultrasound guidance**: Using real-time imaging to ensure accurate injection placement

Footnote Summary

- Injections can reduce pain, inflammation, or nerve irritation
- PRP may support healing in chronic injuries
- Steroids work quickly but aren't for repeated use
- Imaging guidance improves safety and accuracy
- Always discuss risks and benefits with your provider

Neuromodulation for Chronic Foot & Ankle Pain

When surgery is not possible or not wanted

- Some foot and ankle pain is caused by irritated or damaged nerves. When medications, therapy, bracing, and injections have failed — and surgery is not the right option — **neuromodulation** may help.
- Neuromodulation uses a gentle electrical signal to "quiet" nerve pain. These minimally invasive procedures are done through small skin openings, with no large incisions.

What Are the Options?

There are two main types of neuromodulation used for chronic foot and ankle pain:

1. Peripheral Nerve Stimulator (PNS)

Targets one nerve, one location

Best for:

- Pain in one specific part of the foot or ankle
- Nerve pain following an injury or surgery
- Pain that follows the path of a single nerve
- Patients who cannot take strong pain medications

How it works:

- A small wire (lead), about the size of angel hair pasta, is placed near the painful nerve.
- You "test" the device for 1 week to see if it improves your pain.
- If helpful, a permanent version is implanted under the skin for long-term use.

How it helps: The stimulator sends gentle electrical pulses that calm nerve activity and reduce pain signals.

2. Dorsal Root Ganglion (DRG) Stimulation

Best for more widespread or complex pain

Best for:

- Nerve pain involving most of the foot or leg
- Widespread or radiating pain
- **CRPS** (Complex Regional Pain Syndrome)
- Patients not candidates for major surgery

How it works:

- Leads are placed near the **dorsal root ganglion** — a nerve cluster in the lower spine.
- You try the device for 1 week. If it helps, you proceed to permanent placement (leads + battery).

How it helps: Calms nerve pain at the source, especially for burning, tingling, electric shock pain, or extreme skin sensitivity.

Notes:

Who Might Benefit from Neuromodulation?

Neuromodulation may help you if:

- You have chronic **nerve pain** in the foot or ankle
- You **do not want** or **cannot undergo surgery**
- Other treatments haven't helped
- You are dealing with **post-surgical nerve pain**
- You want to reduce your need for medication

⚠ These procedures **do not fix bones or tendons**, but they can **reduce nerve-related pain** and help you move better with less discomfort.

Key Terms

- **Corticosteroid**: A medication used in injections to reduce inflammation and pain
- **CRPS (Complex Regional Pain Syndrome)**: A chronic nerve pain condition that sometimes follows injury or surgery
- **DRG (Dorsal Root Ganglion)**: A group of nerves in the lower spine that transmit pain signals from the legs and feet
- **Nerve block**: A targeted injection that numbs a nerve to reduce or diagnose pain
- **PNS (Peripheral Nerve Stimulator)**: A small implanted device that calms a specific painful nerve using gentle electrical pulses
- **PRP (Platelet-Rich Plasma)**: A regenerative treatment using your own blood to support healing
- **Tendon sheath**: The protective sleeve around a tendon, often inflamed in tendonitis
- **Ultrasound-guided**: A method that uses ultrasound to help place injections or leads accurately

Notes:

Footnote Summary

- Neuromodulation is a non-surgical option for people with nerve-related foot and ankle pain that hasn't improved with other treatments.
- PNS helps with pain in one area; DRG helps with widespread nerve pain.
- These devices don't fix structural issues but can reduce nerve pain and improve daily comfort.
- Ask your provider if you're a candidate for a neuromodulation trial.

Notes:

SECTION 6

Prevention & Foot Health Maintenance

Daily habits that strengthen your feet and protect against injury.

Daily Foot Care

Simple habits that protect your feet every day

- Your feet carry you thousands of steps each day. Daily care helps prevent pain, injuries, and infections—especially if you have diabetes, neuropathy, or circulation issues.
- These small habits can make a big difference over time.

1. Wash and Dry Your Feet Daily

- Use warm (not hot) water and mild soap
- Dry well, especially **between the toes**
- Helps prevent fungus, blisters, and skin irritation
- If you can't reach your feet, use a long-handled sponge or ask for help

2. Check Your Feet Every Day

Look for:

- Redness
- Cracks or cuts
- Swelling
- Color changes
- New calluses or blisters
- Nail changes

Daily checks are essential if you have:

- Diabetes
- Neuropathy
- Circulation problems
- Limited vision or mobility

Notes:

3. Moisturize (But Not Between Toes)

- Apply lotion to tops, bottoms, and heels
- Avoid between the toes to prevent excess moisture

Best options:

- Thick creams
- Urea based creams for cracked heels

4. Trim Toenails Safely

- Cut **straight across**, not too short
- Smooth sharp edges with a file.

Don't cut your own nails if you have:

- Diabetes
- Poor vision
- Difficulty reaching your feet

5. Wear Clean, Breathable Socks

- Change daily
- Choose socks that:
    - Fit well
    - Wick away moisture
    - Are seamless if you have sensitive skin

Best materials:

- Cotton blends
- Moisture-wicking athletic socks

6. Choose Supportive Footwear Every Day

Even indoors, supportive shoes reduce injury and fatigue. Look for:

- Arch support
- A firm heel
- A wide toe box
- Cushioning

Avoid:

- Flat flip-flops
- Worn-out shoes
- High heels
- Thin soles

7. Rotate Your Shoes

Alternate shoes daily to let them dry fully

Helps prevent:

- Odor
- Moisture buildup
- Fungus
- Pressure points

8. Manage Calluses & Dry Skin Gently

Do not cut calluses at home.

- Use a pumice stone or foot file
- Moisturize afterward
  See a podiatrist if calluses are painful, thick, or cracking

9. Protect Your Feet in Public Places.

Wear sandals or flip-flops in:

- Gyms
- Hotel showers
- Locker rooms
- Public pools

Helps prevent:

- Athlete's foot
- Warts
- Toenail fungus

10. Care for Your Heels

Dry, cracked heels can split and lead to infection. Help them heal by:

- Soaking feet 5–10 minutes
- Gently filing thick skin
- Applying thick heel cream at night
- Wearing socks afterward

11. When to Call Your Provider

Seek care if you notice:

- Redness or swelling that lasts more than a few days
- Pain that doesn't improve
- Cracks or sores that won't heal
- Sudden numbness or tingling
- Signs of infection (warmth, pus, odor)

This is especially important if you have **diabetes or neuropathy**.

Key Terms

- **Callus**: Thickened skin caused by rubbing or pressure
- **Fungus**: Germs that thrive in warm, moist places and can cause athlete's foot or nail infections
- **Heel fissure**: A deep crack in the heel that may bleed or become infected
- **Ingrown nail**: When the edge of a toenail grows into the skin, causing pain or swelling
- **Moisture-wicking**: Fabric that draws sweat away from the skin to keep feet dry

Notes:

Footnote Summary

- Wash, dry, check, and moisturize your feet daily
- Trim toenails straight across and avoid lotion between toes
- Wear clean socks and supportive shoes—even at home
- Protect feet in public spaces and call your provider for redness, swelling, or non-healing sores

Nail Care & Ingrown Toenail Prevention

Building on your daily foot care routine

Toenails may seem small—but when things go wrong, they can cause big problems. Painful ingrown nails, infections, and nail damage are common in people with tight shoes, poor circulation, diabetes, or reduced sensation in the feet. Good nail care is a simple but powerful way to avoid complications.

This section builds on the *Daily Foot Care* habits by focusing specifically on **toenails**—how to protect them, trim them, and spot early warning signs of trouble.

1. Trim Toenails Properly

The most important tip: **Trim nails straight across.**
Avoid rounding the corners or cutting them too short, which increases the risk of ingrown toenails.

Quick recap of safe trimming:

- Cut straight across
- Leave a small margin—do not cut to the quick
- Smooth rough edges with a nail file
- Avoid digging into the nail sides

If you're unsure or have trouble seeing or reaching your nails, ask a podiatrist for help—especially if you have diabetes or neuropathy.

2. Keep Nails Clean and Dry

This is covered in your daily routine but is especially important for nail health.
After bathing:

- Dry thoroughly under and around each nail
- Avoid letting moisture collect under nail edges
- Change damp socks quickly

This helps prevent:

- **Fungal infections**
- **Bacterial infections**
- **Athlete's foot that spreads to the nails**

3. Use Proper Tools — and Don't Pick or Rip

Only use **clean, sharp nail clippers** designed for toenails (wider and flatter). Never rip, peel, or bite at nails.

This helps avoid:

- Splits
- Nail lifting
- Nail bed infections

Clean clippers with rubbing alcohol after each use.

4. Support Your Nails with the Right Shoes

Shoes that are too tight or narrow **can trigger ingrown nails** and nail bruising (black toenails).

Choose:

- Wide toe boxes
- Breathable material
- Room for your toes to move

Avoid:

- Pointy shoes
- High heels
- Old or worn-out shoes that compress your toes

5. Recognize Early Signs of Nail Trouble

Don't try to "dig out" an ingrown toenail at home. This often causes **worsening pain or infection.**

Warning signs:

- Pain along the edge of the nail
- Redness or swelling
- Warmth or pus
- Skin growing over the nail edge

6. When to See a Specialist

See a podiatrist for regular nail care if you have:

- **Diabetes**
- **Neuropathy**
- **Thick or curved nails**
- **Vision or mobility limitations**
- **Repeated ingrown toenails**

Key Terms

- **Cuticle**: The thin layer of skin at the base of the toenail that protects against infection
- **Fungus**: Germs that grow in warm, moist places and can infect nails or skin
- **Ingrown toenail**: When the nail edge grows into the surrounding skin, causing pain and inflammation
- **Nail plate**: The hard, visible part of the nail
- **Toe box**: The front area of a shoe where the toes rest; too-narrow toe boxes increase nail pressure

Footnote Summary

- Proper nail care prevents many painful conditions.
- Trim toenails **straight across**, keep them **clean and dry**, and **wear shoes that fit well**.
- Avoid home removal of ingrown nails—see a specialist, especially if you have diabetes or reduced feeling in your feet.

Choosing Proper Footwear

Shoes that support your feet, reduce pain, and prevent injury

Wearing the right shoes is one of the **best things you can do** to protect your feet and ankles. Good shoes reduce pressure, improve balance, support your arches, and help prevent common problems like heel pain, bunions, and tendonitis.

This guide shows what to look for—and what to avoid.

1. Why Shoe Choice Matters

Poor footwear is linked to:

- Heel and arch pain (like plantar fasciitis)
- Bunions and hammertoes
- Tendonitis and stress injuries
- Ankle sprains

Your feet absorb thousands of steps a day. Supportive shoes reduce strain and keep your joints aligned.

Notes:

2. What to Look for in a Supportive Shoe

Feature	What It Does	What to Look For
Wide toe box	Prevents pressure on toes	Room to wiggle, rounded shape
Firm heel counter	Stabilizes heel	Back of shoe should feel stiff
Arch support	Supports flat or high arches	Built-in support or room for inserts
Cushioning	Absorbs shock	Not too soft or thin
Stiff sole (bend test)	Reduces strain	Shoe should bend only at the toes
Breathable material	Reduces sweat and irritation	Mesh, knit, or leather uppers

🩺 *Surgeon's tip: Test the shoe while standing. If it feels unstable or rubs, it won't get better with time.*

3. How to Check the Fit

- **Length:** Leave a thumb's width between your longest toe and the end
- **Width:** Toes should not feel squeezed or numb
- **Walk Test:** Shoes should feel good right away—not after "breaking in"
- **Try on shoes late in the day:** Feet swell by evening
- **Bring orthotics if you wear them**

4. Match Shoes to Your Foot Type

Foot Type	Look For	Avoid
Flat feet	Motion-control shoes, arch support	Soft, unsupportive soles
High arches	Good cushioning, soft insoles	Hard, rigid shoes
Bunions or wide feet	Wide toe box, soft material	Pointy or narrow shoes
Diabetes or neuropathy	Seamless interior, cushioned sole	Barefoot walking, tight spots
Achilles pain	Slight heel lift or wedge	Completely flat shoes

Helps with:

- Flat feet
- Plantar fasciitis
- Tendon issues (especially posterior tibial tendon)

5. Shoes to Avoid

Avoid these unless you have zero foot issues:

- Flip-flops and ballet flats
- High heels
- Shoes that pinch or squeeze
- Very soft soles with no support
- Worn-out shoes
- Shoes with no arch support

6. When to Replace Shoes

- **Every 6–12 months** (or 300–500 miles for walkers/runners)
- Replace if you notice:
    - Worn-out soles
    - Flattened cushioning
    - Uneven wear
    - Pain returning

Key Terms

- **Arch support**: Helps hold up your arch and reduce strain
- **Breathable material**: Fabric that allows airflow to reduce sweat
- **Heel counter**: The stiff back part of a shoe that holds the heel stable
- **Motion-control shoe**: Built for people with flat feet or overpronation
- **Toe box**: The front of the shoe where your toes sit; wide is better

Footnote Summary

- Choose shoes with **support, cushioning, and a wide toe box**
- Avoid flimsy shoes or ones that pinch
- Try shoes **on later in the day**, walk on hard floors, and **replace them regularly**

Notes:

Fall Prevention & Safe Walking Habits

Simple ways to stay steady, confident, and injury-free

Falls are one of the **most common causes of foot and ankle injuries**. But most falls can be prevented with smart habits, better shoes, and a few home changes.

Why Fall Prevention Matters.

Simple changes can prevent most falls. A fall can lead to:

- Sprains and fractures
- Chronic pain
- Slower healing
- Fear of walking
- Loss of independence

You're at higher risk if you have:

- Balance or vision problems
- Neuropathy or arthritis
- Muscle weakness
- A history of falls
- Age-related changes
- Instability
- Neuropathy
- A recent injury
- Fear of falling

Notes:

Top Fall Prevention Tips

At Home

- **Clear walkways:** Remove clutter, loose rugs, cords, pet toys
- **Improve lighting:** Use nightlights, bright bulbs, and motion sensors
- **Dry floors:** Clean up spills and use non-slip mats in bathrooms and kitchens
- **Use handrails and grab bars:** Install them on stairs and in bathrooms

Footwear

- Wear **supportive, well-fitting shoes** with good tread
- Avoid flip-flops, loose slippers, socks-only walking, and worn-out shoes

Walking Safety

- Move slowly when getting out of bed or a chair
- Keep your **head up, eyes forward**
- Take short, even steps
- Use a **cane or walker** if your provider recommends it
- Avoid carrying heavy or bulky items that block your view or throw off balance

Build Balance & Strength

Simple daily exercises can greatly reduce fall risk:

- Stand on one leg (hold a counter)
- Heel-to-toe walking
- Chair stands (sit to stand)
- Gentle ankle mobility and weight shifting

These strengthen your feet, ankles, hips, and core.

Surgeon's tip: "A flexible Achilles helps stabilize your foot tripod—big toe, little toe, and heel."

When Outside

- Watch for uneven pavement
- Walk in daylight or well-lit areas
- Use handrails on stairs or ramps
- Wear sturdy, grippy shoes
- Be cautious on sand, wet surfaces, or ice

When to Talk to Your Provider

Let your provider know if you have:

- Frequent stumbles
- Recent falls
- Dizziness
- Numbness in your feet
- Fear of walking alone
- Sudden changes in strength or balance

Key Terms

- **Assistive device**: Cane or walker that improves stability
- **Balance**: Staying steady while walking or standing
- **Fall risk**: The chance of tripping, slipping, or losing balance
- **Posture**: How you carry your body while walking or standing
- **Tread**: The grip or traction on the bottom of a shoe

Footnote Summary

- Keep walkways clear, wear supportive shoes, and improve lighting
- Practice balance and strength exercises daily
- Use handrails and assistive devices when needed
- Tell your provider if you've fallen, feel unsteady, or notice numbness

Diabetes & Foot Safety

Protecting your feet when you have diabetes

Diabetes can reduce **feeling** (neuropathy) and **blood flow** (poor circulation) to your feet. This makes it easy to miss small injuries—and harder for them to heal.

But here's the good news: **Daily foot care and early attention can prevent most serious problems.**

Why Diabetes Affects the Feet

1. **Neuropathy** (nerve damage)
   You may not feel pain, cuts, heat, or pressure—so small injuries go unnoticed.

2. **Poor Circulation**
   Less blood flow = slower healing, higher infection risk, and increased chance of ulcers.

Essential Daily Habits

(*These are covered in more detail in the Daily Foot Care section—review if needed!*)

- ☐ Check your feet every day
  Look for redness, swelling, blisters, cracks, color changes, drainage, or open areas. Use a mirror, phone, or ask for help if needed.
- ☐ Wash & dry daily
  Use warm (not hot) water and dry between your toes.
- ☐ Moisturize (but not between toes)
  Prevents cracked skin. Use thick or urea-based creams.
- ☐ Trim nails carefully
  Straight across, not too short. Never dig at corners. If you have trouble, see a podiatrist.

- ☐ Always wear shoes
  Even indoors. Choose well-fitted, cushioned shoes or diabetic slippers. Never go barefoot.
- ☐ Never self-treat calluses
  Use a pumice stone gently. See a podiatrist for thick or cracked areas.
- ☐ Protect from heat and cold
  Don't use heating pads, hot water bottles, or test bath water with numb feet.

Choose Footwear Designed for Diabetes

Look for:

- Extra depth
- Soft, smooth lining
- Wide toe box
- Arch support
- Room for inserts or orthotics

More details in the Choosing Proper Footwear section.

When to Call Your Provider

Even **minor problems can become serious fast** in people with diabetes.

Call your provider or podiatrist if you notice:

- A blister, cut, or sore that doesn't improve in 1–2 days
- Redness or warmth
- Swelling
- Drainage or odor
- Skin that turns black, blue, or feels cold
- Sudden numbness or pain

Get Regular Foot Exams

- At least **once a year**
- Every **3–6 months** if you've had ulcers or neuropathy
- A podiatrist can safely trim nails, treat calluses, and check circulation

Control Blood Sugar = Healthier Feet

Keeping blood sugar in your target range:

- Protects nerves
- Improves circulation
- Speeds healing
- Lowers your risk of infection

Key Terms

- **Callus**: Thickened skin caused by rubbing or pressure—can hide sores underneath
- **Circulation**: Blood flow through the body; poor circulation slows healing
- **Neuropathy**: Nerve damage causing numbness, tingling, or burning in the feet
- **Podiatrist**: A medical foot and ankle specialist
- **Ulcer**: An open sore that doesn't heal normally and can become infected

Footnote Summary

- Check your feet daily and never ignore changes
- Keep your skin clean, dry, and moisturized
- Wear protective, well-fitting shoes at all times
- Report cuts, sores, or swelling right away
- Work with a podiatrist and keep your blood sugar stable

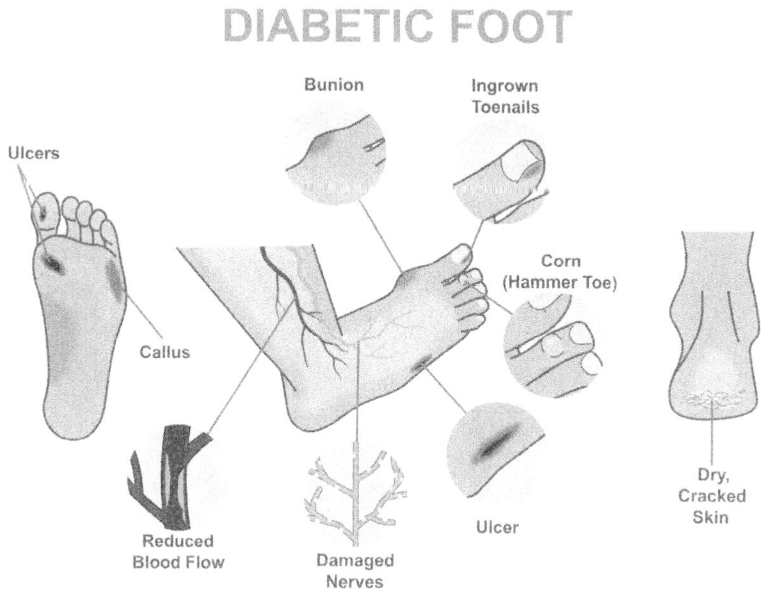
DIABETIC FOOT
Bunion
Ingrown
Toenails
Ulcers
Corn
(Hammer Toe)
Callus
Reduced
Blood Flow
Damaged
Nerves
Ulcer
Dry,
Cracked
Skin

Notes:

SECTION 7

Living With Ankle & Foot Pain

Tools to stay active and manage chronic symptoms confidently.

Pacing & Activity Modification

Staying active while protecting your feet

You don't have to stop moving just because of foot or ankle pain—**but how you move matters**.

By adjusting how much, how often, and how intensely you move, you can stay fit while giving your feet the rest they need.

What Is Pacing?

Pacing means spreading out your activity so you don't overload painful joints or healing tissue.

■ Do enough to stay strong
❌ Avoid overdoing it and triggering flare-ups

Pacing helps:

- Reduce pain and swelling
- Avoid overuse
- Support healing
- Keep you active—but in control

Simple Pacing Tips

- **Break tasks into chunks** (e.g. 20 min activity → rest → 20 min more)
- **Alternate standing and sitting** throughout the day
- **Rest before pain starts**—don't wait until your foot is throbbing
- **Use a timer** to change position every 20–30 min

Notes:

Safer Ways to Stay Active

You can still exercise without making symptoms worse.

Best Low-Impact Options

- Swimming or water aerobics
- Stationary or recumbent bike
- Elliptical or rowing (light intensity)
- Seated strength training
- Gentle yoga or Pilates

These support:

- Circulation
- Muscle strength
- Heart health
- Mental well-being

Ask your provider when it's safe to resume regular workouts.

Avoid During Flare-Ups

❌ Running, jumping, high-impact sports
❌ Long hikes or fast-paced walking
❌ Prolonged standing on hard floors

Protect Your Feet at Home & Work

(Refer back to Fall Prevention, Footwear, and Daily Foot Care for detailed tips.)

Standing Safety

- Sit every 20–30 minutes
- Wear supportive house shoes—not bare feet on hard floors
- Use cushioned mats in kitchens or work areas
- Shift weight often—don't lock knees

Smart Walking

- Start with short, flat-surface walks
- Wear well-fitted, supportive shoes
- Avoid uneven ground and rushing

Workplace Adjustments

- For standing jobs:
    - Anti-fatigue mats
    - Compression socks (if approved)
    - Scheduled breaks
- For walking jobs:
    - Rotate tasks
    - Stretch often
    - Reduce walking during flare-ups
- For desk jobs:
    - Keep feet flat and supported
    - Avoid crossing legs
    - Change positions often

Small Home Changes That Help

- Clear clutter and cords
- Add night lights
- Use handrails on stairs
- Keep daily items easy to reach
- Use a shower chair during recovery if needed

Notes:

Protecting Your Feet Long-Term

Consistency matters more than intensity. Healthy feet come from smart habits.

DO:

- Wear supportive shoes every day
- Stretch calves and arches regularly
- Strengthen ankles and feet
- Replace worn-out shoes
- Moisturize your feet
- Check for changes, especially with diabetes or neuropathy

AVOID:

- Barefoot walking on hard floors
- High heels or narrow shoes
- Long periods of standing
- Sudden increases in activity
- "Pushing through" pain

Key Terms

- **Activity modification**: Changing how you move to reduce symptoms
- **Anti-fatigue mat**: A cushioned mat to reduce pressure when standing
- **Flare-up**: A short-term worsening of pain or swelling
- **Low-impact exercise**: Movement that avoids stress on joints (e.g. swimming, cycling)
- **Pacing**: Spreading activity throughout the day to avoid overload

Notes:

Footnote Summary

- Pacing and low-impact activity protect healing feet
- Break tasks into chunks and rest before pain starts
- Use supportive shoes, cushioned mats, and smart walking habits
- Small changes at home and work help reduce foot stress
- Consistent movement—not overdoing it—is key to long-term foot health

Notes:

SECTION 8

When Surgery Is Needed

Understanding surgical choices and what to expect during recovery.

How Surgeons Decide

Understanding when surgery is the right choice—and when it isn't

Not everyone with foot or ankle pain needs surgery. In fact, most conditions improve with non-surgical care like therapy, braces, injections, footwear changes, and activity modification.

Surgeons recommend surgery only when:

- Other treatments haven't worked
- The problem is interfering with your life
- Surgery has a good chance of helping you
- You are willing to do the hard work of therapy after surgery

And surgery is always a **shared decision** — you and your surgeon make the plan together.

Surgery Is Usually the Last Step

Most chronic foot and ankle problems are treated without surgery first. This might include:

- Physical therapy
- Supportive footwear or orthotics
- Injections or anti-inflammatory medications
- Bracing or boot use
- Activity or weight modification
- Casting or immobilization

Surgeon's note: "Your foot will take time to heal — you get to decide if that happens now, or later when it might take even longer."

What Surgeons Look At

Foot surgeons consider many factors—not just your scans.

1. Your Symptoms

- How bad is the pain?
- Does it affect walking, balance, work, sleep, or daily life?
- Do you feel unstable or unsafe on your feet?

2. How Long It's Been a Problem

Most new injuries don't need surgery. Chronic problems (lasting 6–12 months or longer) may require stronger treatment.

3. What You've Already Tried

Before recommending surgery, your surgeon checks if:

- Therapy was done properly
- Bracing, footwear, or orthotics were used
- Medications and injections were given time to work
- You've tried changing your activities or weight-bearing

4. Imaging That Matches the Problem

Surgeons use imaging (like X-rays or MRIs) to **confirm**, not just diagnose.
They look for alignment problems, tendon damage, arthritis, or fractures that **match your symptoms**.

5. How It Affects Your Daily Life

Surgery may be more likely if the problem affects:

- Walking or standing
- Work or caregiving
- Hobbies or exercise
- Driving, sleeping, or balance

Notes:

6. Your Overall Health

Some conditions affect healing. Your surgeon will talk with you about:

- Diabetes
- Circulation problems
- Smoking
- Medications
- Weight
- Other medical conditions

Sometimes, surgery is delayed until these are better controlled.

When Surgery Is Needed Sooner

Some conditions **should not wait**, including:

- Displaced fractures
- Tendon ruptures (like Achilles tears)
- Progressive deformities
- Severe infections or deep wounds
- Unstable ankle injuries

These problems may worsen without early surgical repair.

When Surgery Is NOT a Good Option

Your surgeon may advise **against** surgery if:

- The pain is mild or manageable
- Imaging doesn't explain your symptoms
- Non-surgical treatments haven't been fully explored
- Surgery would not likely help
- The risks outweigh the benefits
- The problem is mostly cosmetic
- The recovery would be longer or harder than the benefit

Making the Final Decision: Together

Good surgeons practice **shared decision-making**. They'll talk honestly with you about:

- The **realistic** benefits of surgery
- The risks involved
- What recovery will require (e.g., crutches, boots, therapy)
- Whether your goals match what surgery can offer

Your Goals Matter

Surgery is about improving your quality of life. Tell your surgeon what matters most to you. Common goals include:

- Walking without pain
- Returning to work or sports
- Wearing normal shoes
- Sleeping better
- Regaining balance or confidence
- Preventing deformity

Key Terms

- **Deformity**: A change in the foot's shape or alignment that can cause pain or limit movement
- **Imaging**: Diagnostic tools like X-rays, MRIs, or ultrasound
- **Instability**: When a joint feels loose or gives out during movement
- **Non-surgical treatment**: Care options like therapy, braces, and medication
- **Shared decision-making**: You and your surgeon work together to choose the best path forward

Notes:

Footnote Summary

- Most foot and ankle problems get better without surgery
- Surgery is only recommended when other treatments fail and symptoms significantly impact your life
- Your overall health, goals, imaging, and daily function all play a role
- You and your surgeon decide together, based on what's safest and most helpful for you

Notes:

Types of Foot & Ankle Surgery

What's done, why it helps, and how it supports healing

Foot and ankle surgeries are carefully chosen to treat specific problems—like torn tendons, painful arthritis, fractures, deformity, or nerve issues.

You won't need to memorize medical terms. But understanding what each type of surgery aims to fix can help you feel more informed and confident.

1. Joint Surgeries: When the problem is inside the joint

These surgeries help when cartilage wears out, joints get inflamed, or bones don't move properly.

A. Arthroscopy ("Scope Surgery")

- A tiny camera and tools are inserted through small cuts
- Used to clean up scar tissue or remove loose pieces inside the joint

Helps with:

- Mild arthritis
- Ankle impingement
- Cartilage injuries
- Swelling that hasn't responded to other care

**Small incisions, faster healing, less pain afterward*

Notes:

B. Fusion (Arthrodesis)

- Two bones are joined permanently to stop painful movement
- The joint no longer bends, but it becomes stable

Helps with:

- Severe arthritis
- Instability
- Foot deformities
- Chronic pain that hasn't responded to treatment

**Pain is reduced because the joint no longer grinds*

Common fusion areas: Big toe, midfoot, subtalar joint, ankle

C. Joint Replacement (Arthroplasty)

- Damaged joint surfaces are removed and replaced with artificial parts
- Keeps the joint moving while reducing pain

Helps with:

- Severe ankle arthritis
- Patients who want to preserve movement
- Not recommended for everyone — depends on bone quality, age, and activity level

**Less pain with continued joint motion*

2. Tendon Surgeries: When tendons are torn or inflamed

Tendons connect muscle to bone. Surgery helps restore strength, stability, or motion.

Notes:

A. Tendon Repair

- Torn ends are stitched back together

Used for:

- Achilles tears
- Peroneal tendon tears
- Posterior tibial tendon injuries

B. Tendon Debridement

- Damaged, thickened, or irritated tissue is removed

Used for:

- Chronic tendonitis
- Scar tissue
- Overuse injuries

C. Tendon Transfer

- A healthy tendon is moved to do the job of a weak or damaged one

Used for:

- Severe flatfoot
- Loss of function
- Balance or walking problems due to tendon weakness

**Improves motion and support*

3. Bone Surgeries: When bone alignment or healing needs correction

These surgeries help when bones are out of position, broken, or putting pressure in the wrong spots.

A. Osteotomy (Bone Cut + Reposition)

- Bone is carefully cut and moved into a better position

Used for:

- Bunions
- Hammertoes
- Flatfoot or high arches

**Relieves pain and restores proper alignment*

B. Fracture Fixation

- Broken bones are repositioned and held in place with screws, plates, or pins

Used for:

- Unstable or shifted fractures
- Breaks that won't heal on their own

**Speeds healing and helps prevent deformity*

4. Soft Tissue Surgeries: When ligaments, fascia, or nerves are involved

A. Ligament Repair or Reconstruction

- Tightens or rebuilds stretched-out ligaments

Used for:

- Chronic ankle sprains
- Feeling of instability

**Prevents future sprains and improves balance*

Notes:

B. Plantar Fasciitis Surgery

- A small cut is made in the tight plantar fascia to release tension

Used for:

- Severe plantar fasciitis that hasn't improved with therapy

**Relieves heel pain when nothing else works*

C. Nerve Surgeries

- Either remove a nerve mass (like a Morton's neuroma)
- Or free a compressed nerve (like tarsal tunnel release)

Used for:

- Burning or shooting pain
- Numbness
- Nerve entrapment

**Helps restore sensation and reduce nerve irritation*

5. Deformity Corrections: For toes, arches, and alignment

These surgeries aim to realign bones and improve foot shape.

A. Bunion Correction

- Realigns the bones around the big toe
- Often includes bone cut and soft tissue repair

**Improves shoe fit, reduces pain, and prevents crowding*

B. Hammertoe Correction

- Tight tendons are released
- Joints may be straightened or fused

**Eases pressure and helps fit into shoes*

C. Flatfoot Reconstruction

- Combination of tendon repair, bone cuts, and ligament tightening
- Rebuilds the arch and corrects ankle position

**Improves stability and walking comfort*

Minimally Invasive Options

Not every surgery needs large cuts. Some procedures can be done through **tiny incisions**, such as:

- Minimally invasive bunion correction
- Hammertoe straightening
- Small tendon repairs

**Smaller scars, faster healing, and less pain — if you're a candidate*

Key Terms

- **Arthroscopy**: Surgery done through small incisions using a camera
- **Debridement**: Removal of damaged or irritated tissue
- **Fixation**: Screws or plates used to hold bones in place
- **Fusion**: Permanently joining two bones to stop painful motion
- **Osteotomy**: Cutting and shifting a bone to improve alignment

Footnote Summary

- Foot and ankle surgeries are **designed for specific problems**, like torn tendons, arthritis, or deformities
- Your surgeon chooses a procedure based on your **symptoms**, **function**, and **goals**
- Options range from **minimally invasive procedures** to **realignment, fusion, or tendon repair**
- Surgery is meant to **reduce pain**, **improve stability**, and **help you move better**

Common Foot & Ankle Problems and the Surgeries That Help

Problem	Possible Surgeries
Arthritis (Ankle, Foot, Toe)	• Arthroscopy (clean-up) • Joint Fusion • Joint Replacement (ankle only)
Tendon Tears or Tendonitis	• Tendon Repair • Tendon Debridement • Tendon Transfer
Flatfoot or Arch Collapse	• Flatfoot Reconstruction • Tendon Transfer • Osteotomy (bone cut)
Bunion or Hammertoe	• Bunion Correction • Hammertoe Correction • Osteotomy
Instability / Sprains	• Ligament Repair or Reconstruction
Plantar Fasciitis	• Partial Plantar Fascia Release
Nerve Pain / Compression	• Neuroma Removal • Tarsal Tunnel Release
Fracture That Won't Heal	• Fracture Fixation with screws or plates
Severe Deformity	• Osteotomy • Joint Fusion • Flatfoot Reconstruction

Notes:

Surgical Risks, Benefits, Expectations

What to know before having foot or ankle surgery

Foot and ankle surgery can significantly improve pain, alignment, and mobility — but it also requires preparation, patience, and a clear understanding of risks and recovery.

This section explains the **benefits**, **risks**, **what to expect before and after surgery**, and how you can take an active role in your recovery.

Benefits of Surgery

No surgery creates a "perfect" foot, but it can provide lasting relief and better movement.

Common benefits include:

- Less pain
- Improved walking and balance
- Better foot alignment
- Greater mobility and independence
- Better shoe fit
- Less swelling or instability
- Prevention of deformity getting worse

For some, surgery offers the best path back to:

- Work
- Hobbies or sports
- Normal daily activities

Risks of Surgery

All surgeries carry some risk. Your surgeon will talk through your specific risks and help reduce them.

Common risks:

- Pain
- Swelling
- Bruising
- Stiffness
- Slow healing

Less common risks:

- Infection
- Nerve irritation or numbness
- Blood clots
- Wound healing issues
- Reaction to anesthesia
- Hardware irritation (screws or plates)
- Need for additional surgery
- Limited joint motion

Risks may be higher if you have:

- Diabetes
- Poor circulation
- Neuropathy
- Smoking history
- Autoimmune disease
- Obesity

Before Surgery: How to Prepare

Pre-Op Appointment

- Review your symptoms and surgical plan
- Discuss risks, benefits, and goals
- Get instructions about medications and mobility tools (boot, crutches, etc.)

Medical Clearance

- You may need bloodwork, an EKG, or clearance from your doctor—especially if you have heart disease, diabetes, or take multiple medications

Home Setup

- Create a rest area with essentials in reach
- Prepare meals in advance
- Arrange help for children, pets, or chores
- Add grab bars, nightlights, or a shower chair if needed

Mobility Tools

- You may be prescribed a:
  - Walking boot
  - Knee scooter
  - Crutches or cane
  - Post-op shoe

Medication Instructions

- You may need to:
  - Stop NSAIDs or blood thinners
  - Take specific medications the morning of surgery
  - Avoid food or drink after a certain time

What to Expect on Surgery Day

Before surgery:

- Check-in and health review
- IV is started
- Meet your anesthesia team
- Surgical site is marked

During surgery:

- You receive anesthesia (general or sedation)
- The surgical team completes your procedure

After surgery:

- Your foot is wrapped and elevated
- You're monitored for pain and comfort
- You may go home the same day

Recovery Expectations

Healing is a process—it depends on your health, the type of surgery, and how well **you follow your plan**.

Pain

- Most patients have pain for a few days
- You may be prescribed pain medication and anti-inflammatories
- Ice and elevation help reduce discomfort

Weight-Bearing

- Some surgeries allow early walking
- Others require 2–8 weeks of no weight-bearing
- You may need a boot, scooter, or crutches

Swelling

- Can last weeks to months
- Elevate your foot above heart level for 20–30 minutes, several times a day

Wound Care

- Keep dressings clean, dry, and intact
- Don't remove wraps unless instructed

Follow-Up Visits

- Your surgeon or PA/NP will:
  - Check incision healing
  - Remove stitches (usually around 10–14 days)
  - Adjust walking restrictions
  - Review X-rays
  - Start physical therapy

Physical Therapy

- Helps restore:
  - Flexibility
  - Strength
  - Swelling control
  - Balance and walking
  - Return to daily activity

Returning to Activities *(Typical ranges vary by procedure):*

- Desk work: 1–3 weeks
- Standing or walking jobs: 4–12 weeks
- Driving: when cleared
- Light exercise: 6–12 weeks
- Running/sports: 3–6 months
- Full healing: 6–12 months

Your Role in Recovery

What you do after surgery is just as important as what happens in the OR.

Support healing by:

- Following instructions exactly
- Using your boot or brace
- Elevating often
- Not smoking
- Controlling blood sugar (if diabetic)
- Attending all follow-ups and physical therapy

Common Healing Timelines

- Soft tissue swelling: 3–6 months
- Tendon healing: 3–12 months
- Bone healing: 8–12 months
- Nerve healing: months to years (varies widely)
- Plantar fasciitis: slow, but steady with consistency

Key Terms

- **Fusion**: A surgery that joins bones to stop painful movement
- **Incision**: The surgical cut made during surgery
- **Mobility devices**: Tools like crutches, a scooter, or cane used after surgery
- **Physical therapy**: Exercise-based rehab that restores motion and strength
- **Pre-Op / Post-Op**: The periods before and after surgery
- **Weight-bearing**: How much pressure you're allowed to put on your foot

Footnote Summary

- Surgery can relieve pain, improve motion, and help you return to daily life
- All surgeries have risks—your team works to keep you safe
- Prepare your home and body before surgery
- Recovery takes time—expect rest, therapy, and restrictions
- Good recovery depends on following your surgeon's instructions

Notes:

SECTION 9

Mobility Aids & Home Equipment

Tools that make daily activities easier while you heal.

The Basics of Devices

What helps you move safely during recovery

After foot or ankle surgery, the right tools can make daily life easier and safer. This section covers the most common devices and how to prepare your home for healing.

Mobility Devices

Crutches

- Keep weight off the injured foot
- Best for short distances
- Require good balance and arm strength
- Use padding to protect underarms

Walker

- Most stable option
- Ideal for people who feel unsteady
- Helps prevent falls
- Allows slow, steady movement

Cane

- Used only when some weight-bearing is allowed
- Hold in the hand **opposite** the injured foot
- Assists with balance, not full support

Knee Scooters

- Great alternative to crutches
- Keeps foot off the ground, knee rests on padded base
- Better for longer distances
- Not ideal for stairs or uneven ground
- Best for longer non-weight-bearing recovery

Walking Boots vs. Cast

Your provider will choose what's safest based on your condition.

Walking Boot (CAM Boot)

- Removable (ask when it's safe to remove)
- Adjustable straps
- Can be walked in if cleared by your provider
- Can shower without it
- May need a shoe lift on the other foot to keep hips level

Cast

- Not removable
- Maximum protection
- Keeps the foot completely still
- Must be kept dry at all times
- Often used for fractures or strict healing protocols

Helpful Home Equipment

Shower Chair

- Sit safely during showers
- Prevents slipping
- Essential for non-weight-bearing patients

Bedside Commode

- Useful if getting to the bathroom is difficult
- Reduces fall risk at night

Notes:

Setting Up Your Home

- Clear walkways of clutter
- Remove throw rugs
- Install night lights in hallways
- Use non-slip mats in kitchen and bathroom
- Keep essentials within reach (water, medications, phone)
- Place a chair in the shower
- Arrange for help with pets, meals, and laundry
- Keep your boot/scooter/crutches by the bed for nighttime use

Cast & Splint Care

- Keep it dry (cover for showers, never submerge)
- Do **not** stick anything inside to scratch
- Do **not** cut or trim the cast
- Elevate your foot to reduce swelling
- Watch the skin around the edges for irritation

Call Your Surgeon Immediately If:

Circulation Problems

- Toes turning blue, purple, or very pale
- Toes that feel cold or lose sensation

Nerve Problems

- New numbness or tingling
- You can't move your toes

Compartment or Pressure Problems

- Pain suddenly worsens, even with medication
- Cast feels like it's "crushing" or "pinching"

Wet or Damaged Cast

- Wet or Damaged Cast
- Foul odor or soft spots
- Cracks or broken sections

Home setup for healing checklist

- ☐ Nightlights in bedroom and hallways
- ☐ Remove throw rugs and clutter
- ☐ Block pets from running underfoot
- ☐ Keep supportive shoes and mobility aids nearby
- ☐ Place chair in shower for stability
- ☐ Store essentials within arm's reach
- ☐ Keep your walking boot near the bed for bathroom trips

When to call your surgeon

- Pain suddenly gets worse
- New coldness, numbness, or discoloration in toes
- Your boot causes rubbing or skin sores
- Swelling increases again after improving
- You hear or feel a "pop"
- You suddenly can't put weight on the foot
- A cast, brace, or boot breaks or becomes loose

Footnote Summary

- Crutches, walkers, canes, and knee scooters help protect your foot while keeping you mobile
- Boots are removable (with guidance); casts are not and must stay dry
- Set up your home to reduce fall risks and make daily tasks easier
- Call your provider if you have sudden pain, numb toes, or a damaged cast

Notes:

SECTION 10

Mindfulness & Natural Pain Management

Supporting your body and mind through chronic or persistent pain.

Calming your body, protecting your mind, and supporting healing

Foot and ankle pain affects more than just your joints — it also impacts your **nervous system, sleep, mood, and daily life**.

This section offers simple, natural ways to **support healing, reduce pain, and calm the body**.

Why It Matters

- Chronic pain makes your nervous system more sensitive
- Stress and poor sleep make pain worse
- Calming techniques help your brain and body "reset"
- Natural strategies don't replace medical care—but they **enhance recovery**
- Many tools are free, simple, and can be practiced at home

Mental health & chronic pain

- Living with foot or ankle pain can affect more than your body
- It can change how you move, how you sleep, and even how you feel emotionally
- And the reverse is also true: your stress, mood, and worry can change how your body feels pain

Pain and the Mind Body Connection

- Stress can make small pain feel bigger
- Tense muscles = tighter tendons and stiffer joints

Tools That Help Calm the Nervous System

Deep Breathing Techniques

1. The 4–6 Breath
Inhale through your nose for 4 seconds → Exhale for 6 seconds
Repeat for 10–15 breaths
**Lowers tension and sharp pain*

2. Box Breathing

Inhale → Hold → Exhale → Hold (4 seconds each)

**Helps focus and calm a racing mind*

3. Belly Breathing

Place one hand on belly → Breathe so belly rises

**Reduces shallow "stress breathing"*

Guided Imagery

- Close your eyes and picture a calming scene
- Use all senses: sights, sounds, smells
- Stay in the scene for 1–3 minutes

**Helps turn down pain signals*

Progressive Muscle Relaxation (PMR)

- Tense each muscle group for 3 seconds, then fully relax
- Start at your feet and move upward

**Releases stored muscle tension*

Pain Journaling

Track your symptoms and triggers daily. Include:

- Pain level (0–10)
- What you were doing
- What helped or worsened pain
- Mood or stress level
- Sleep quality

**Helps identify flare-up patterns and guide better choices*

Notes:

When Fear of Pain Causes More Pain

- Avoiding all movement can lead to:
  - Weak muscles
  - Reduced balance
  - Stiff joints
- **Safe, gentle movement is almost always helpful**
- Your provider will tell you what is safe

Reducing Overuse of Pain Medications

Overuse of meds can cause:

- Stomach irritation (NSAIDs)
- Liver strain (acetaminophen)
- Tolerance or dependence (opioids)
- Rebound pain

Healthier habits:

- Use medicine only as prescribed
- Pair with ice, elevation, stretching, rest
- Try topicals like Voltaren or lidocaine
- Use breathing during flare-ups
- Pace your activities

Sleep: A Natural Pain Reliever

Pain and poor sleep go hand in hand. Healing happens during sleep.

Better Sleep Tips:

- Keep a regular bedtime
- Avoid screens 1 hour before bed
- Keep your bedroom cool and dark
- Use pillows to support your foot
- Do gentle stretches or breathing before bed

If pain wakes you up:

- Reposition with pillows
- Try breathing or calf stretches
- Use ice (if cleared by your provider)

How to Break the Stress-Pain Cycle

Pain → Stress → Tension → More Pain

What stress does:

- Tightens muscles
- Increases inflammation
- Makes pain feel sharper
- Worsens sleep
- Triggers shallow breathing

What helps:

- Deep breathing
- Gentle stretching
- Heat on tense muscles (if cleared)
- Journaling
- Short walks or light movement
- Mindfulness, prayer, or guided imagery
- Talking to a supportive friend or counselor

Key Terms

- **Guided imagery**: Relaxing by imagining peaceful scenes
- **Mindfulness**: Calmly focusing on the present moment
- **Pain journaling**: Writing down symptoms and patterns
- **Progressive muscle relaxation**: Tensing then relaxing muscles to ease tension
- **Stress response**: The body's physical reaction to fear, worry, or pressure

Footnote Summary

- Pain affects both body and mind—natural tools help both
- Breathing, stretching, and journaling lower pain sensitivity
- Stress makes pain worse—relaxation helps break the cycle
- Good sleep, gentle movement, and pacing support long-term healing
- Mind-body tools work best when practiced consistently—not just during flare-ups

Notes:

SECTION 11

Tracking Worksheets

Tools to help you stay organized, monitor progress, and prepare for your next visit

- Tracking your symptoms, care routines, and questions can make your appointments more helpful and can speed up recovery
- These worksheets give you a simple way to notice patterns, remember details, and stay on top of your treatment plan
- You can print these pages, copy them into a notebook, or rewrite them in your own style

Pain Diary (Daily or Weekly)

Date: ____________________________

Pain Level (0–10): ____________________________

Where is the pain located?

☐ Heel
☐ Arch
☐ Toes
☐ Ankle
☐ Outside foot
☐ Inside foot
☐ Top of foot
☐ Other: __________________________

Describe the pain:

☐ Sharp
☐ Dull
☐ Achy
☐ Burning
☐ Tingling
☐ "Stabbing"
☐ Numbness

What was I doing when pain started?

____

What made it better?

- ☐ Rest
- ☐ Ice
- ☐ Heat
- ☐ Stretching
- ☐ Boot or brace
- ☐ Medication
- ☐ Elevation
- ☐ Other: ______________________

What made it worse?

- ☐ Walking
- ☐ Standing
- ☐ Stairs
- ☐ Exercise
- ☐ Barefoot
- ☐ Certain shoes
- ☐ Work duties
- ☐ Other: ______________________

Notes:

Symptom Tracker (Weekly Summary)

Week of: ______________________________

Symptoms I Felt This Week

Check all that apply:
- ☐ Swelling
- ☐ Bruising
- ☐ Stiffness
- ☐ Numbness
- ☐ Tingling
- ☐ Weakness
- ☐ Instability (“giving way”)
- ☐ Locking or clicking
- ☐ Pain at night
- ☐ Pain first thing in the morning

Overall Change This Week:
- ☐ Better
- ☐ Worse
- ☐ No change

Notes:

Medication Log *(Track what you take, how much, and whether it helps.)*

Medication Name: ____________________________

Dose: ____________________________

Time Taken: ____________________________

Reason for Taking It:

☐ Pain
☐ Swelling
☐ Nerve pain
☐ Post-surgery
☐ Other ________________________

Did it help?

☐ Yes
☐ No
☐ Somewhat

Any side effects?

☐ None
☐ Upset stomach
☐ Drowsiness
☐ Dizziness
☐ Constipation
☐ Other: ________________________

Notes:

Post-Surgery Milestones *(A simple checklist to track recovery progress.)*

My Surgery Date: ________________________

Early Recovery (Weeks 1–2)

☐ Pain improving
☐ Swelling improving
☐ Incision clean and dry
☐ Taking medications as directed
☐ Keeping weight off foot (if instructed)
☐ Using boot or cast correctly

Middle Recovery (Weeks 3–8)

☐ Cleared for partial weight-bearing
☐ Started gentle motion
☐ Pain becoming less sharp
☐ Boot fitting well
☐ Starting to regain strength

Later Recovery (Weeks 8–12+)

☐ Cleared for full weight-bearing
☐ Starting physical therapy
☐ Improvement in walking
☐ More stable and confident
☐ Returning to daily routines

Long-Term Recovery (3–12 Months)

☐ Strength improving
☐ Swelling mostly gone
☐ Walking longer distances
☐ Resuming exercise (as allowed)
☐ Meeting personal goals

Questions for Your Next Visit *(Write down anything you want to remember.)*

Questions About Symptoms

- ☐ What is causing my pain?
- ☐ Is this normal for my stage of healing?
- ☐ Are my symptoms improving as expected?

Questions About Activity

- ☐ When can I go back to work?
- ☐ When can I drive again?
- ☐ What types of exercise are safe for me now?
- ☐ How should I pace my activities?

Questions About Treatment

- ☐ Is my boot or brace still needed?
- ☐ Should I continue ice or heat?
- ☐ Do I need physical therapy?
- ☐ Are there other treatments I should consider?

Questions About Surgery (If relevant)

- ☐ How long will recovery take?
- ☐ What risks apply to me?
- ☐ What can I expect in the first 2 weeks?
- ☐ What should I avoid doing?

My Personal Questions:

1. ____________________
2. ____________________
3. ____________________
4. ____________________

Notes:

GLOSSARY (A–Z)

A

- **ABI (Ankle-Brachial Index)** — A simple test that compares blood pressure in the arm and ankle to check blood flow.
- **Achilles Tendon** — The strong tendon at the back of the ankle that connects the calf to the heel.
- **Acetaminophen** — A medicine that reduces pain but not swelling.
- **Acute Pain** — New pain that starts suddenly, usually after an injury.
- **Activity Modification** — Changing how you move to reduce pain or protect an injury.
- **Adult-Acquired Flatfoot** — Arch collapse that develops later in life.
- **Anti-Fatigue Mat** — A soft mat that reduces strain when standing for long periods.
- **Anti-Inflammatory** — A medication or treatment that reduces swelling and irritation.
- **Antifungal** — Medicine that treats fungal infections.
- **Arch** — The curved middle part of the foot that helps absorb shock.
- **Arch Support** — A shoe feature or insert that helps support the arch.
- **Arthritis** — Joint wear and swelling that cause pain and stiffness.
- **Arthrodesis (Fusion)** — A surgery that joins two bones so they no longer move.
- **Arthroplasty (Joint Replacement)** — A surgery that replaces a worn-out joint with artificial parts.
- **Arthroscopy** — A type of surgery that uses a small camera and tools through tiny incisions.
- **Assistive Device** — A tool like a cane or walker that helps with balance or safety.
- **At-Home Care** — Simple treatments you do yourself, like stretching, rest, or proper shoes.

B

- **Balance** — The ability to stay steady while standing or walking.
- **Balance Training** — Exercises that improve stability and help prevent falls.
- **Ball of the Foot** — The area just behind the toes where pressure increases when walking.
- **Blistering** — Small fluid-filled bubbles on the skin.
- **Bone Spur** — Extra bone that forms from pressure or arthritis.
- **Brace** — A support worn to protect the foot or ankle.
- **Breathable Material** — Fabric that lets air in and sweat out.
- **Bunion** — A bump at the base of the big toe that forms when the toe shifts outward.
- **Bunionectomy** — A surgery to correct a bunion by realigning bone and soft tissue.
- **Burning Pain** — Hot, tingling pain often caused by irritated nerves.

C

- **Callus** — Thickened skin from pressure or rubbing.
- **Calf Muscle** — Muscle in the back of the leg that helps you walk.
- **Calf Stretch** — A gentle stretch that loosens the calf and reduces tendon strain.
- **Cartilage** — Smooth tissue that cushions joints.
- **Cast** — A hard shell that keeps bones from moving so they can heal.
- **Cheilectomy** — Surgery to remove bone spurs from the big toe joint.
- **Chronic Pain** — Pain lasting longer than three months.
- **Circulation** — Blood flow through the body.
- **Compression** — Gentle pressure used to reduce swelling or support joints.
- **Crutches** — Mobility aids that help keep weight off an injured foot.
- **CT Scan** — A special X-ray test that shows detailed pictures of bones.

- **Custom Orthotics** — Shoe inserts made specifically for your foot.
- **Cuticle** — The thin skin at the base of the nail that protects it from infection.
- **Cyst** — A small fluid-filled bump under the skin.

D

- **Debridement** — Trimming or removing damaged or thickened tissue.
- **Deformity** — A change in the normal shape of the foot or toes.
- **Diabetic Foot** — Foot problems caused by diabetes, like numbness or slow healing.
- **Diabetic Shoes** — Special shoes that reduce pressure and prevent wounds.
- **Dislocation** — When a bone slips out of place.
- **Dorsiflexion** — Bending the foot upward toward the shin.
- **DRG (Dorsal Root Ganglion Stimulator)** — A device that targets nerves in the lower back that send pain into the foot.

E

- **Edema** — Swelling caused by fluid buildup.
- **Elevation** — Raising the foot above your heart to reduce swelling.
- **Extension** — Straightening a joint.
- **Excessive Pronation** — When the foot rolls too far inward while walking.

F

- **Fascia** — Strong tissue that supports the arch of the foot.
- **Fissure (Heel Fissure)** — A deep crack in the heel.
- **Fixation** — Screws, plates, or pins used to hold bones in place while they heal.
- **Flare-Up** — A temporary increase in pain or swelling.
- **Flatfoot** — When the arch is low or collapsed.

- **Foot Drop** — Weakness that causes the toes to drag while walking.
- **Fracture** — A broken bone.
- **Fungus** — Germs that grow in warm, moist environments.
- **Fusion** — See Arthrodesis.

G

- **Gait** — The way you walk.
- **Guided Imagery** — Relaxing by imagining calm scenes or places.

H

- **Hallux** — The big toe.
- **Hammertoe** — A toe bent upward in the middle like a hammer.
- **Heel Counter** — The firm back part of a shoe that stabilizes the heel.
- **Heel Lift** — A pad placed in the shoe to reduce Achilles strain.
- **Heel Spur** — A small piece of extra bone under the heel.
- **High Arch (Cavus Foot)** — A foot with a very high arch.

I

- **Immobilization** — Keeping the foot still with a cast, boot, or brace.
- **Impingement** — Pinching of soft tissue inside a joint.
- **Imaging** — Tests like X-ray, MRI, CT, or ultrasound that show bones or soft tissues.
- **Ingrown Toenail** — When the nail grows into the skin.
- **Inflammation** — Redness, swelling, warmth, or irritation.
- **Instability** — A joint that feels wobbly or may give out.
- **Insertional Tendonitis** — Irritation where a tendon attaches to bone.

J

- **Joint** — Where two bones meet.
- **Joint Space** — The gap between bones filled with cartilage.

K

- **Knee Scooter** — A rolling device you kneel on to avoid putting weight on your foot.

L

- **Lacquer** — A medicated nail polish for fungus treatment.
- **Lateral** — The outer side of the foot or ankle.
- **Ligament** — Strong tissue that connects bones.
- **Low-Impact Exercise** — Gentle movement that protects joints.

M

- **Metatarsal Pad** — A soft pad that relieves pressure behind the toes.
- **Metatarsals** — The long bones behind the toes.
- **Mobility** — How well your joints move.
- **Mobility Devices** — Tools like crutches, scooters, or walkers that help you move safely.
- **Motion-Control Shoe** — A shoe for flat feet or overpronation.
- **MRI** — A scan that shows detailed pictures of soft tissues.
- **Mulder Click Test** — A test for Morton's neuroma.
- **Muscle Relaxation** — Tightening and releasing muscles to reduce tension.
- **Moisture-Wicking Fabric** — Fabric that pulls sweat away from the skin.

N

- **Nail Plate** — The hard top part of the nail.
- **Nerve Block** — An injection that numbs a nerve.
- **Neuroma** — A thickened, irritated nerve.
- **Neuropathy** — Nerve damage causing numbness or burning.
- **Night Splint** — A device that stretches the foot while you sleep.
- **Non-Weight-Bearing** — Not putting weight on the foot.

O

- **Offloading** — Shifting pressure away from a painful area.
- **Orthopedic Surgeon** — A doctor who treats bones and joints.
- **Orthotics** — Shoe inserts that support the foot.
- **Overuse Injury** — Pain from doing too much activity too quickly.
- **Osteotomy** — Cutting and repositioning a bone.

P

- **Pacing** — Spreading activities out to avoid flare-ups.
- **Pain Journaling** — Writing down symptoms to find patterns.
- **Partial Nail Removal** — Removing just the part of the nail causing problems.
- **Peroneal Tendons** — Tendons on the outside of the ankle.
- **Physical Therapy (PT)** — Exercise-based rehabilitation.
- **Plantar Fascia** — Thick tissue on the bottom of the foot.
- **Plantar Fasciitis** — Inflammation of the plantar fascia.
- **PNS (Peripheral Nerve Stimulator)** — A device that calms pain signals in one nerve.
- **Posterior Tibial Tendon** — Tendon on the inside of the ankle that supports the arch.
- **Pronation** — Inward roll of the foot while walking.
- **Progressive Muscle Relaxation** — Tightening and relaxing muscles to reduce stress.
- **PRP (Platelet-Rich Plasma)** — Treatment using part of your own blood.

Q

- **Quality of Life** — How pain affects daily activities and mood.

R

- **Radiculopathy** — Pain from a pinched nerve in the spine.
- **Range of Motion** — How far a joint can move.
- **RICE** — Rest, Ice, Compression, Elevation.
- **Rocker-Bottom Sole** — A curved shoe sole that helps the foot roll forward.
- **Rupture** — A significant tear in a tendon.

S

- **Scaling** — Dry, flaky skin.
- **Shared Decision-Making** — When patients and providers choose a plan together.
- **Single-Leg Heel Raise** — A test of posterior tibial tendon strength.
- **Shoe Tread** — The grip on the bottom of a shoe.
- **Splint** — A removable support that keeps a joint still.
- **Sprain** — An injury to a ligament.
- **Stabilization** — Keeping a joint from moving too much.
- **Stress Fracture** — A tiny crack in a bone from overuse.
- **Strengthening** — Exercises that build muscle.
- **Supination** — Outward roll of the foot.
- **Suture** — Stitches used to close a wound.
- **Swelling** — Fluid buildup that makes an area look larger or feel tight.

T

- **Tendon** — Tissue that connects muscle to bone.
- **Tendon Sheath** — The sleeve that helps a tendon glide.
- **Tendon Tear** — A partial or full rip of a tendon.
- **Tendonitis** — Swelling or irritation of a tendon.
- **Tinel's Sign** — Tapping over a nerve to check for irritation.
- **Toe Box** — The front part of a shoe where the toes sit.
- **Toe Spacer** — A soft device that separates toes to reduce rubbing.
- **Turf Toe** — A sprain of the big-toe joint.

U

- **Ulcer** — A sore that doesn't heal well.
- **Ultrasound** — Imaging that uses sound waves to view soft tissue.
- **Ultrasound-Guided Injection** — An injection done with ultrasound to place medicine accurately.

V

- **Valgus/Varus** — Inward tilt (valgus) or outward tilt (varus) of a foot or joint.
- **Vascular** — Related to blood vessels.

W

- **Walking Boot (CAM Boot)** — A removable boot that limits ankle motion.
- **Weight-Bearing** — How much weight you are allowed to put on your foot.
- **Wound Care** — Keeping a cut or incision clean and healing.

X

- **X-ray** — A picture that shows bones and joint spaces.

Y

(No common foot or ankle terms beginning with "Y.")

Z

- **Z-Lengthening** — A surgery that lengthens a tight tendon using a Z-shaped cut.

Author Note

As a Physician Assistant, educator, and long-time clinician in spine and musculoskeletal medicine, my mission is simple: **to make medical information clear, compassionate, and truly useful.**

Foot & Ankle Pain 101: A Patient's Complete Guide to Symptoms, Treatments, and Prevention was written for anyone who has struggled to find straightforward answers about foot and ankle pain — one of the most common, frustrating, and often misunderstood categories of orthopedic problems.

Foot and ankle pain affects everything: balance, walking, sleep, work, and even confidence.

Patients deserve explanations that make sense.

This book joins my growing Patient Education 101 series, which includes **Knee Pain 101, Hip Pain 101, Shoulder Pain 101, Chronic Neck Pain 101**, and other guides designed to help patients understand what is happening in their bodies. My experience in **interventional spine and pain management**, along with earlier years assisting in **lower-extremity surgeries**, has given me a unique perspective on how closely connected the foot, ankle, and spine really are — and how much relief comes from understanding the "why" behind a symptom.

Every book in this series is written for real people — patients, caregivers, and families — who want clear, accurate information without medical jargon. You'll find practical explanations, simple drawings, checklists, and step-by-step tools that you can use before, during, and after your appointments.

Spanish-language editions are pending to reach more North American readers and ensure vital medical education is accessible to everyone.

Each book in this series uses trusted U.S. medical guidelines (AAOS, UpToDate, NIH, and major U.S. hospital systems such as Mayo Clinic and Johns Hopkins). Content is reviewed periodically to keep information accurate and current.

If this book brings you clarity, comfort, or confidence in your health journey, then it has done its job.

You are stronger than you think — from the ground up.

— **Stacie the PA**
Duke Residency Trained Physician Assistant
Founder, Stacie the PA via *Medical Things Explained*
Author, *Patient Education 101 Series*

📚 More Helpful Books

by Stacie the PA

Clear, compassionate, and practical guides written by a medical provider who cares.

💓 Hypertension 101
Understand high blood pressure and how to manage it — simply.

🦵 Knee Pain 101
From anatomy to treatment options, a complete patient reference.

🦴 Hip Pain 101
Everything you need to know about hip pain, diagnosis, and care.

🦴 Osteoporosis 101
A clear, supportive guide to bone loss, prevention, and treatment options.

💪 Shoulder Pain 101
An easy-to-follow guide to common shoulder problems and solutions.

🧠 Neck Pain 101
A step-by-step look at spine-related neck pain, diagnosis, and treatment options.

💧 Kidney Stones 101
A simple guide to causes, treatments, and prevention strategies.

🫁 Pneumonia 101
Learn the basics of prevention, symptoms, and recovery.

🔥 Gout 101
Practical answers about causes, flares, and long-term care.

🦠 **Diverticulosis 101**
Understand symptoms, triggers, and treatment of this common digestive condition.

🎗 **Breast Cancer 101: A Patient's Complete Guide to Symptoms, Treatments, and Prevention**
A compassionate, evidence-based guide for patients, survivors, and caregivers — covering everything from diagnosis to recovery and long-term wellness.

🎗 **Cáncer de Mama 101: Guía Completa para Pacientes**
The Spanish-language edition of *Breast Cancer 101* — designed for North American Spanish-speaking patients and families with the same supportive, educational approach.

✷ **Menopause 101: What Every Husband Should Know About the Change**
A practical guide that bridges understanding and communication between partners.

🦶 **Foot & Ankle Pain 101** *(this book)*
Understand the most common causes of foot and ankle pain — and the treatments that help.

✷ **Coming Soon:** Hand and Arm Pain 101, Sciatica 101.

Visit **StaciethePA.com** or find my author page on Amazon under **"Stacie the PA."**

Made in the USA
Monee, IL
04 November 2026

67378699R00154